Skills Manual
for Introduction
to Person-Centered
Nursing

Skills Manual for

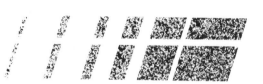

Introduction to Person-Centered Nursing

Janice B. Lindberg, *R.N., M.A., Ph.D.*

Former Area Chairperson, Fundamentals
Associate Professor
The University of Michigan, School of Nursing
Ann Arbor, Michigan

Mary Love Hunter, *R.N., M.S.*

Clinical Nursing Specialist
University of Michigan Hospitals
Coordinator, Fundamentals
Assistant Professor
The University of Michigan, School of Nursing
Ann Arbor, Michigan

Ann Z. Kruszewski, *R.N., M.S.N.*

Assistant Professor, Fundamentals
The University of Michigan, School of Nursing
Ann Arbor, Michigan

J.B. Lippincott Company Philadelphia

London   Mexico City   New York   St. Louis   São Paulo   Sydney

Sponsoring Editor: Diana Intenzo
Manuscript Editor: Rachel Bedard
Indexer: Ann Cassar
Designer and Art Director: Tracy Baldwin
Production Supervisor: N. Carol Kerr
Production Assistant: J. Corey Gray
Compositor: Monotype Composition Company, Inc.
Printer/Binder: The Murray Printing Company

6 5 4 3 2

The authors and publishers have exerted every effort to ensure that drug selection and
dosage set forth in this text are in accord with current recommendations and practice
at the time of publication. However, in view of ongoing research, changes in
government regulations, and the constant flow of information relating to drug therapy
and drug reactions, the reader is urged to check the package insert for each drug for
any change in indications and dosage and for added warnings and precautions. This is
particularly important when the recommended agent is a new or infrequently
employed drug.

Preface

This skills manual has been designed specifically to accompany the text *Introduction to Person-Centered Nursing*. The volume reflects the authors' belief that technical aspects of professional care also require a person-centered approach. In practice this means that each procedure is accomplished with the person rather than done to him and also that the person's human needs are considered and, indeed, do influence individual modifications of standard procedures. The holistic person remains the object of professional nursing care even though individual procedures concentrate on specific body parts or functions. The need for nursing procedures arises from altered functional abilities; looking beyond the specific altered function, the professional practitioner finds and ministers to the unique holistic individual who is the object of person-centered nursing care.

This manual also reflects the authors' belief that nursing is nursing wherever it happens. Therefore, each procedure is presented with a minimal number of key steps that apply to a variety of circumstances and settings. Only those procedures are presented which, in the authors' opinion, are central to initial professional nursing courses introducing basic skills. In the same spirit, only the physical assessment essential to a specific procedure is presented, either here in brief introductory remarks to that procedure or as a reference to the accompanying text. This approach reflects a different emphasis for presentation of basic procedures.

Janice B. Lindberg
Mary Love Hunter
Ann Z. Kruszewski

Acknowledgments

The authors gratefully acknowledge the many persons who made varied contributions to this laboratory manual. Emily Droste-Bielak, Joan King, Karen Laufer, and Lorraine Wilson, former faculty members at the University of Michigan School of Nursing, contributed to an earlier laboratory manual used within the fundamentals area.

Illustration Credits

Most of the photos in this manual were selected from units of the Lippincott Learning System, a self-instructional audiovisual program. The following units are represented:

Asepsis

* Body mechanics

** Bowel elimination

* Care of the mouth

* Care of the skin

* Making a bed

* Oral medication

* Parenteral medication

* Vital signs

Wound care

** Urine elimination

Respiratory care

A single asterisk indicates units for which the copyright is held by the Regents of the University of Wisconsin/Milwaukee, whose permission to reproduce them here is gratefully acknowledged. A double asterisk indicates that copyrights are held by both the Regents of the University of Wisconsin/Milwaukee and the J.B. Lippincott Co. The absence of an asterisk indicates that the J.B. Lippincott Co. is the sole copyright holder.

Contents

Skills Manual
for Introduction
to Person-Centered
Nursing

Environment

The person who is hospitalized must adapt to activities of daily living (ADL) within an environment which is quite different from that experienced at home. Even the ambulatory person finds that everyday activities like bathing and eating are modified by the hospital environment. Those whose functional abilities are seriously altered may find the hospital environment even more restrictive, especially if they are confined to bed or allowed limited freedom. Additionally, the usually uneventful routines like bathing may become lengthy procedures.

Further, because of the number of persons living in close proximity in a hospital setting, the risk of cross infections between patients and staff members is an ever present danger that must be managed with environmental controls. Some of these controls are the direct responsibility of the nurse and will be detailed under the headings of medical and surgical asepsis. These environmental procedures vary in complexity from handwashing to strict isolation techniques involving surgical gowns and gloves. All are intended to minimize the risk of cross infection and thereby protect individuals who might otherwise be at risk.

The basic principles underlying asepsis and environmental safety apply not only to the hospital environment but to the home environment as well. Nurses should be alert to client needs which suggest that instruction about ways to control environmental hazards may be helpful.

Medical Asepsis

When carrying out nursing activities, you will be aware of a great emphasis on safety. One of the important responsibilities you will have as a nurse is to control the spread of infection. To participate properly in this aspect of nursing care, it is important that you understand some of the basic principles of medical asepsis.

Infections are caused by microorganisms. Those microorganisms that produce disease are called *pathogens*. Pathogens may be spread in a variety of ways, for example, direct contact, body discharges, food, air, and so on.

Usually healthy people are protected from pathogenic invasion by basic hygiene practices and by natural body defense mechanisms. However, hospitalized persons may have lowered defenses because of age and illness or because of possible contact with new microorganisms to which they have no immunity. Because of this, nurses must always be concerned with disease control.

There are two kinds of aseptic techniques practiced in the hospital—medical and surgical. The term *surgical asepsis* is often used to mean free from *all* microorganisms; *medical asepsis* means free from *pathogenic* microorganisms.

Certain terms used in relation to medical and surgical asepsis are often used interchangeably and are therefore confusing. When an item is spoken of in terms of surgical asepsis, it is either sterile (uncontaminated) or unsterile (contaminated). When it is spoken of in terms of medical asepsis, it is either clean (free of pathogens) or dirty (carrying pathogens).

```
       Surgical asepsis              Medical asepsis
          /      \                      /      \
     Sterile   Contaminated         Clean    Dirty
```

For now we will center our discussion on medical asepsis. There are some general practices that must be observed if one is to provide a medically aseptic environment for hospitalized persons.

One of the most common means by which pathogenic microorganisms are carried and transmitted is by the hands. Therefore, hands should be washed frequently but especially before handling food, before eating, after using a handkerchief, after going to the toilet, and before and after each client contact.

Other aspects of personal hygiene should be observed: fingernails should be cleaned frequently and kept neatly trimmed; rings, if worn, should be smooth so as not to harbor microorganisms or scratch others; a watch should have an expansion band so that it can be pushed up onto the forearm while the hands are being washed; and long hair should be tied back neatly to prevent transfer of microorganisms.

In addition to handwashing and personal hygiene, certain other practices help ensure a safe environment. It is important to keep constantly in mind what is "clean" and what is "dirty." For example, soiled linen or other items should be carried in such a way that they do not touch the uniform. When brushing or scrubbing articles, clean away from yourself. Clean least soiled areas first, then the more soiled ones. Dispose of soiled or used items directly into appropriate containers, and pour soiled liquids directly into the drain to avoid splashing.

Keeping the hands clean and providing a safe environment depend on the reliability of each person. Effective practice of medical asepsis is up to each member of the hospital staff.

Although most procedures involve principles of medical asepsis, specific procedures that apply to this concept include the following:

- Handwashing
- Bedmaking
- Isolation

Handwashing

Objective

The student will be able to do the following:

1 Wash hands according to principles of medical asepsis.

Procedure for Handwashing

Key Steps	Discussion
Stand in front of sink with knees slightly bent and with soap and water controls within easy reach.	Good body mechanics prevent strain.
Roll sleeves above elbows, and remove watch. (If watch has expansion band, move it well toward elbow.)	

Key Steps	*Discussion*

Turn water on; adjust temperature. (Let water run during entire procedure.)

Warm water removes microorganisms more effectively than cold water, and it removes fewer oils from the skin than hot water.

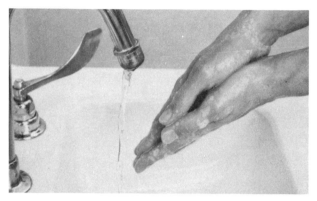

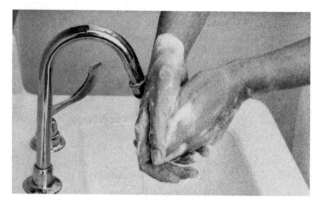

Wet hands, and apply soap; lather well. Rub all surfaces of the hands and fingers for 30 seconds. Pay particular attention to the interdigital areas and fingernails.

Rinse well under running water, keeping hands lower than elbows at all times.

Rubbing and the emulsification of oils on the skin aid in the removal of bacteria.
Microorganism count is higher under nails and between fingers.

Running water aids in the mechanical removal of microorganisms.

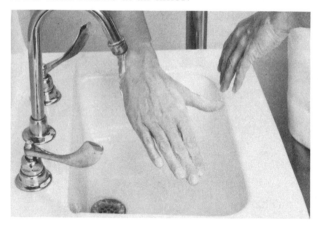

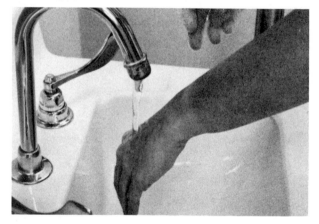

Avoid touching the inner surface of the sink.

Sinks accumulate microorganisms and are considered dirty.

Blot hands; dry thoroughly from fingers to forearms with paper towel.

Microorganisms need moisture to live. Blotting is easier on the skin than rubbing.
Work from most clean to least clean area.

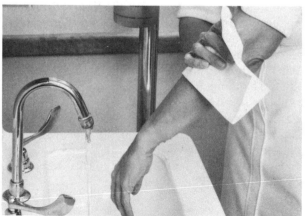

Key Steps

Use dry paper towel to turn off faucet.

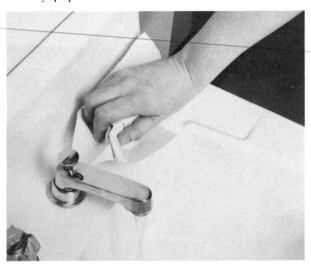

Apply hand lotion if desired.

Discussion

Faucet is contaminated from dirty hand, which turned it on.

Frequent handwashing eliminates natural oils causing dry and cracked skin. Dry, cracked skin is susceptible to bacterial invasion.

Bedmaking

Objectives

The student will be able to do the following:

1 Make a clean and comfortable bed.

2 Protect safety of persons during bedmaking.

3 Use correct body mechanics.

4 Adhere to principles of medical asepsis.

Introduction

The bed is a major object in the environment of the hospitalized person. Even if the person is able to be out of bed much of the day, a comfortable bed contributes to comfort during rest and sleep. For those who must remain in bed for most or all of the time during hospitalization, a comfortable and neat environment is required for all activities of daily living. Careful bedmaking both increases comfort and decreases risk of cross contamination between patients. For many hospitalized persons the bedside will be the only place where they can receive visitors. Therefore, a neat environment may enhance their interactions and increase psychosocial comfort.

Because it is considerably easier to make an unoccupied bed, work should be organized so the bed can be made at times when the person is up and about, perhaps off to an appointment.

When the person must remain in bed, it is best to plan to bathe him, if possible, before fresh linen is provided.

Procedure for Making an Unoccupied Bed

Key Steps

Wash your hands.

Assess need for linen, and gather necessary items. Place them in order of use—the item on top will be used first as follows:

- Mattress pad
- Bottom sheet
- Plastic drawsheet (optional)
- Cotton drawsheet (optional)
- Top sheet
- Blanket
- Spread
- Pillowcase

Raise bed to convenient working height.

Lock wheels of bed; move unneeded furniture out of the way; remove attached equipment (*e.g.,* call light). Put siderails down.

Bring laundry hamper into room, or place empty pillowcase across back of chair for soiled linens.

Remove cases from pillows; place pillows on chair.

Moving around the bed, loosen top and bottom linen from mattress. Avoid shaking linen because fanning soiled linen can spread microorganisms through the air.

Fold in quarters items to be reused (*e.g.,* blanket, spread) and place them across back of chair.

Discussion

Helps avoid the spread of microorganisms.

Saves time—the stack of linen is handled only once.

Lessens back strain.

Uses good body mechanics.

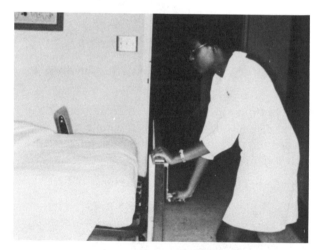

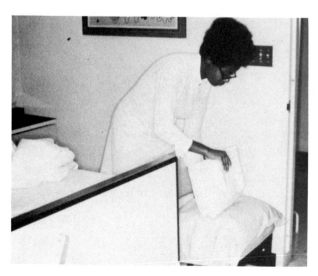

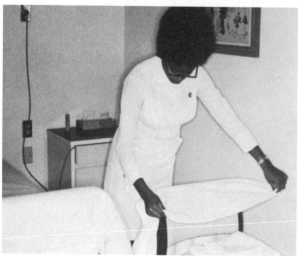

Key Steps

Remove remaining linen and place it in laundry hamper. Do not put soiled linen on floor.

If mattress is to be turned, do so by pulling it toward you and turning it over.
Move mattress to the head of the bed.

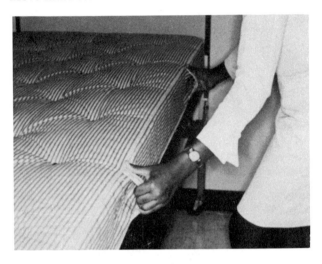

Place mattress pad on mattress and smooth it out.

Place bottom sheet on bed with center fold at the center of mattress and with the seam side of sheet toward the mattress; lower hem should be even with the end of mattress at foot of bed.

Spread sheet, tucking it under at head of bed.

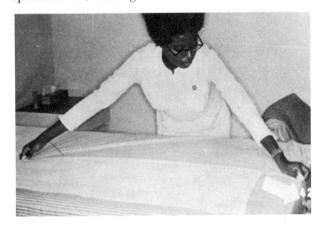

Miter the corner where sheet has been tucked under by doing the following:

- Pick up the side edge of sheet at approximately 10 inches from the head of bed and lay it back over bed, forming a triangular fold.

Discussion

Bed linen harbors microorganisms that can be transferred by direct contact with the nurse's uniform. Placing linens on the floor is unsightly and conducive to the spread of microorganisms.

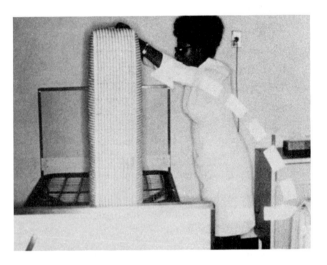

Even small wrinkles may cause irritation, pressure, and skin breakdown.

Completing one side of the bed before moving to the other side saves time and energy.
Rough edges of sheets may be irritating to patients and should be kept away from skin.

Not necessary if fitted bottom sheets are used.

Key Steps

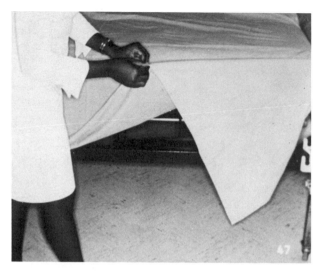

- Place one hand over the fold at the end of the mattress to secure it; with the other hand bring the triangular fold down over it and tuck it under mattress firmly.
- Tuck remaining edge of sheet under mattress.

If a drawsheet is to be used, place it over the middle portion of the bed with the center fold at the center. Tuck the near edge under the mattress securely.

Place the top sheet on bed with center fold at center of bed, seam side up. Align the top edge of sheet with the top edge of mattress. Unfold it toward other side of bed.

Place the spread on bed in the same way as the top sheet.

Make a cuff at the head of bed by folding back the top sheet, and spread approximately 4 inches.

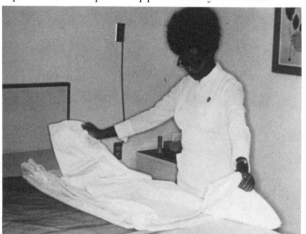

Discussion

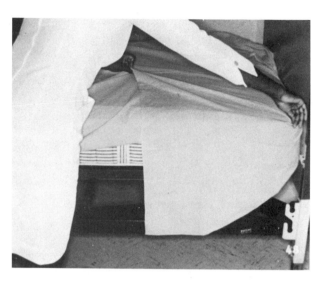

May be used for patients who have draining wounds, who are incontinent, and so forth.

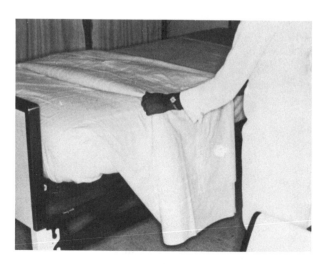

Key Steps

Make a top pleat by folding a 2 inch pleat across the bed about 6 inches from foot of bed. (Use of the pleat in an unoccupied bed is optional.)

Tuck the sheet and spread firmly under mattress at foot of bed.

Miter the corner. Let the side linens hang free.

One side of bed is now completed.

Move to the other side of bed. Straighten bottom sheet and tuck in head edge. Miter the corner.

Working toward foot of bed, pull and tuck the bottom sheet securely.

Discussion

Top linens should not be too tight, because excessive pressure may cause discomfort and poor body alignment, particularly in the lower extremities.

A tight, wrinkle-free foundation lessens discomfort and pressure on the patient.

Pulling the linens to the side and downward, rather than straight across, will keep the mattress in the center of the bed.

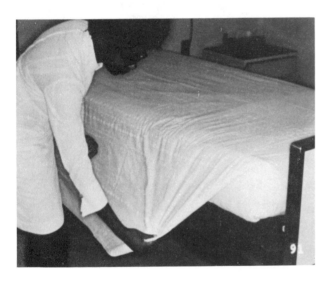

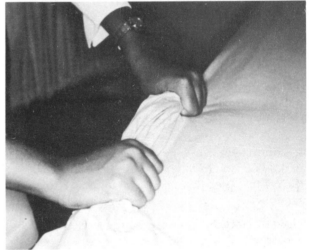

Straighten the drawsheet (if used); pull taut and tuck in securely.

Straighten and tuck the top sheet and spread at foot of bed.

Continue the toe pleat from other side of bed.

Miter the corner. Let side linens hang free.

Fold top sheet over edge of spread.

Remember to use good body mechanics to lessen back strain.

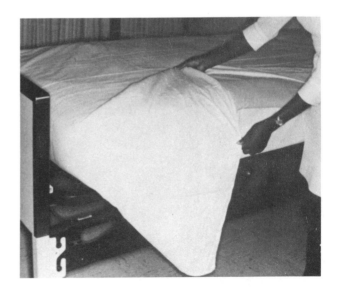

Key Steps

Avoiding contact with uniform, cover pillow with pillowcase as follows:

- Place one hand in center of closed end of pillowcase.
- Gather pillowcase over your hand, inside out.
- Holding pillow with same hand, pull case back over pillow, right side out.

Discussion

Avoids spreading microorganisms.

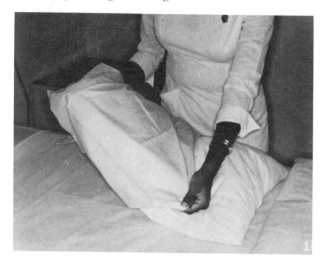

Top bedding may be left up (closed bed) or fan folded back (open bed).

Lower the bed as necessary.
Put call light and bed control within patient's reach.

Replace furniture.

Wash your hands.

An open bed facilitates the patient's return to bed.

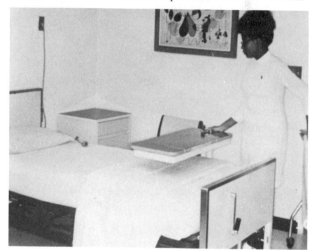

Procedure for Making an Occupied Bed

Key Steps

Inform patient that you are going to change the bed linens. Explain procedure.

Wash hands. Bring necessary linens and linen hamper to bedside.

Remove call light and any other equipment that can be removed.

Raise the side rails, and raise bed to convenient working height.

Discussion

Knowledge of what is going to happen will usually reduce patient's anxiety and increase cooperation.

Avoids unnecessary trips.

Prevents patient from accidentally falling out of bed.

Key Steps	*Discussion*
Place bath blanket over patient, and pull top linens out from underneath. Place soiled linens in hamper.	Protects patient from unnecesssary exposure and chilling.
Roll patient to the far side of bed (the side rail on that side must be up if you are working alone). Adjust pillow as necessary.	Rolling requires less strain on both the patient and nurse.
Loosen linen on vacated side of bed.	
Tuck the soiled linen under patient.	
Place clean bottom sheet on bed. Tuck the sheet under at top, miter the top corner, and tuck the free edge under the mattress to the foot of the bed.	

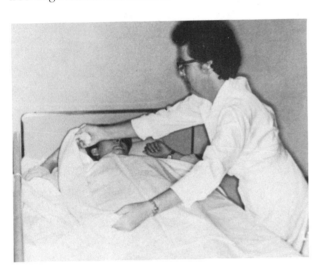

Fan fold the other half of the sheet toward the center of bed, tucking it under the soiled bottom sheet.	
Help the patient to roll over the soiled and fan-folded linen to the clean side of bed. (If working alone, be sure the side rail is up.)	Again, rolling requires less strain on both the patient and nurse.
Remove soiled linen and place in hamper.	
Pull and tuck the bottom linens, as for the unoccupied bed. Pulling linens tightly is more difficult when making an occupied bed.	
Complete top linens as for the unoccupied bed. Remove bath blanket. Adjust pillow. Be sure there is adequate foot room.	
Leave person positioned in comfort and alignment.	
Replace call light. Lower the bed. Raise side rails if necessary. Wash your hands.	Maintains a safe environment at all times.

Modifications

- If the bedridden person tires easily, it may be appropriate to conserve his energy by having someone assist so that the procedure can be accomplished as quickly as possible.

- Hospital beds may be rented or purchased for long-term use at home. If expense is not prohibitive, this convenience may increase comfort for the person and facilitate care for the family. Whether or not a hospital bed will be used at home, family members may be helped to learn bedmaking as a comfort measure.

- The surgical bed is a freshly made bed prepared to receive the postoperative person. It is prepared with one side left open (covers fan folded out of the way) and the top linen not tucked in at the foot. This enables transfer of the postsurgical patient with minimal energy expenditure for patient and staff.

Isolation

Objectives

The student will be able to do the following:

1 State factors involved in the transmission of microorganisms.
2 Describe five types of isolation procedures.
3 Prepare a person and environment for isolation.
4 Put on and remove isolation apparel correctly.
5 Transport an isolated person without contamination.
6 Remove contaminated articles from an isolation unit using principles of medical asepsis.

Isolation procedures are used to protect health-care providers and clients from pathogens and to prevent the transmission of microorganisms. The client may have a communicable disease that requires special techniques to prevent it from being spread to others, or he may have decreased resistance to disease, in which case the goal is to prevent potential pathogens from being transmitted to him.

Understanding the infectious process is essential if isolation techniques are to be carried out correctly. Transmission of pathogens involves the following:

- A causative agent—any pathogen such as bacteria, viruses, fungi, and so on

- A reservoir—a pathogen's normal environment such as food or water

- A mode of escape—a route of exit from the reservoir (*e.g.,* intestinal tract)

- A mode of transfer—a means by which pathogens are spread, such as droplets or direct contact

- A mode of entry—a route of entrance into the body (*e.g.,* respiratory or gastrointestinal tract)

- A susceptible host

Isolation procedures, when properly used, interfere with one of these factors, thus inhibiting the spread of infection.

Categories of isolation and isolation techniques differ according to the hospital and agency because circumstances and facilities vary so much. Generally, isolation policies are planned first to define the categories of conditions requiring isolation and then the procedures necessary for controlling the spread of microorganisms for each category.

Table I-1. Types of Isolation

1. Strict Isolation

- Prevents transmission of all highly communicable diseases spread by both contact and airborne routes.
- The technique requires that the person be in a private room and that anyone coming in contact with the client wear gowns, gloves, and masks and observe strict precautions. All items within the person's unit require special precautions.
- Examples: persons with diphtheria, staphyloccus infections of wounds, smallpox, chickenpox, rabies, and so on

2. Respiratory Isolation

- Prevents the transmission of pathogens by droplet nuclei (coughing, sneezing).
- Requires that the person be in a private room, that masks be worn, and that precautions be taken with respiratory secretions and items contaminated by secretions.
- Examples: persons with tuberculosis, whooping cough, mumps, rubella, and meningococcal meningitis

3. Enteric Isolation

- Prevents diseases that can be transmitted by direct contact or indirect contact with infected fecal material.
- Persons can be cared for safely in a room with others as long as care is taken to avoid fecal contamination.
- Items contaminated by stool or urine require special precautions and disinfection.
- Gowns should be worn by those having direct contact with the person; gloves should be worn only if handling stool or objects contaminated with stool.
- Example: persons with hepatitis, salmonellosis, cholera, typhoid fever, and acute diarrhea with suspected infectious etiology

4. Wound and Skin Isolation

- Prevents cross infection from pathogens transmitted by direct contact with wounds.
- Requires special care of dressings, instruments, and linen that contact wound drainage.
- Anyone coming in contact with drainage should wear gloves and gowns.
- Examples; persons with impetigo, gas gangrene, staphyloccal and generalized wound infections, herpes zoster, and puerperal sepsis–group A streptococci

5. Protective (Reverse) Isolation

- Prevents contact between potential pathogens in the environment and a person with greatly increased susceptibility.
- A private room is necessary. Gowns and masks are worn by anyone entering the room, and gloves are worn by those having direct contact with the person.
- Examples: persons with resistance to infection reduced by extensive burns, immunosuppressive drugs used after transplants, leukemia, bone marrow failure due to radiation therapy, and agranulocytosis

In one approach, diseases are grouped according to what type of isolation precautions are needed, for example:

- Standard
- Strict
- Stool–urine–needle
- Protective

In the other approach, diseases are grouped according to the principal route by which they spread, for example:

- Strict
- Respiratory
- Enteric
- Wound and skin
- Protective

Table I-1 describes this second approach, based on principal route of transmission, and lists briefly both the diseases and general precautions included in each isolation category. Isolation procedure manuals describing institutional policies should be available at each hospital or agency and should be adhered to closely.

Because many isolation procedures require that masks and gloves be worn, that a private room be used, and that the door to the room be closed, the client often feels psychologically as well as physically isolated. The special garb worn by health-care workers may cause him to feel unclean or repulsive. Nurses may spend less time visiting such persons informally because of the effort required to gown and ungown. The person who is so isolated needs sensitive care to help him feel accepted and comfortable within the boundaries of isolation techniques.

Procedure for Preparing a Person and Environment for Isolation

Key Steps

Provide the person to be isolated and family members with necessary information regarding all needs and precautions for the particular isolation.

Hang appropriate isolation card outside the person's door.

Place all necessary isolation supplies in a cart outside the door for easy access.

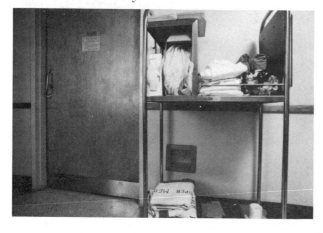

Discussion

Isolation can be a stressful experience for the person and his family. Isolation procedures often produce feelings of loneliness or uncleanliness. Adequate information and support can assist in alleviating anxiety and gaining cooperation.

Isolation cards can be obtained from the U.S. Government Printing Office. Each card briefly lists the precautions for each type of isolation that both personnel and visitors must observe.

If the person requires protective isolation, the cart should be placed inside the person's room. Sterile gowns and gloves may be necessary.
The necessary supplies will vary with each type of isolation. They may include: gowns, masks, gloves, plastic bags for linen and trash, isolation labels, disposable thermometer, disposable stethoscope and blood pressure cuff, and so on.

Key Steps *(italic)* **Discussion**

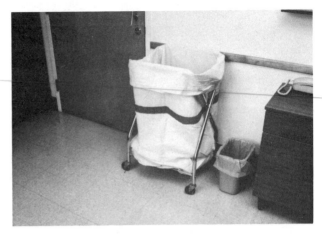

For all isolation procedures except protective, obtain a trash receptacle and linen hamper to place inside the room. Dirty linen and trash are disposed of inside the room to prevent transmitting microorganisms on contaminated articles.

Notify dietary department to prepare meals using disposable trays, dishes, and flatware.

This eliminates the need for double-bagging all the dietary utensils. With disposable items, the entire tray can be discarded in trash receptacle inside the person's room.

Procedure for Donning and Removing Gown, Mask, and Gloves

Key Steps **Discussion**

To put on gown, mask, and gloves:
Remove watch and rings. Secure hair up off shoulders.

If watch is going to be needed in person's room, it should be placed in a plastic bag. This allows for clear view of watch and prevents contamination.

Put gown on. It should overlap well around the back of the uniform and at waist. Tie or secure tabs at neck and waist.

Gowns should be long-sleeved and large enough to sufficiently cover the uniform.
If the gown becomes wet while in direct contact with the person in isolation, it will not provide adequate protection. Change to a dry one immediately.

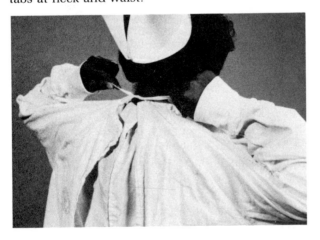

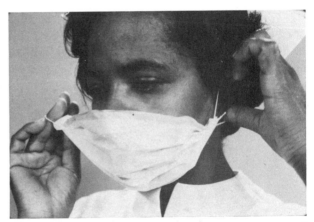

Place mask snugly over nose and mouth and tie strings behind head. Ties should be high enough so that the mask will not slip off.

Most masks will not provide adequate protection if worn longer than 20 minutes because they become damp. Change as frequently as they become damp.

Key Steps

Discussion

Put on gloves, and tuck cuffs of gown into gloves. Gloves should be long enough to cover cuffs of gown. Be sure to change gloves if they are torn while working.

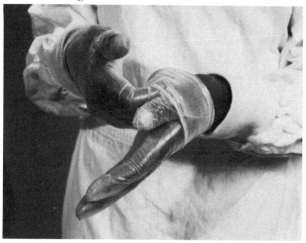

To remove gown, mask, and gloves:
Remaining inside person's room and with gloves on, untie gown at waist.

The contaminated areas of the isolation clothing are the following:

- Front of mask
- Entire front of gown
- The back of gown from waist down
- Waist ties
- Gloves

Remove gloves by pulling them off inside out. Discard them in receptacle near door inside the room. Wash hands immediately.

Hands will probably be contaminated while removing gloves, so careful washing is necessary.

Untie mask, and handling the ties only, discard in receptacle by door inside the room.

Because the front of mask is considered contaminated, care must be taken to only touch ties.
If the person has a highly communicable disease, exceptions may be made to allow masks to be worn until outside of room. Then discard immediately outside in a designated receptacle.

Untie gown at neck. Grasp the gown at shoulders and pull down over arms. Holding gown at shoulders, remove one arm at a time, turning arm of gown inside out as each hand is removed.

The back of the gown from waist to shoulders is considered clean. Therefore, touching the shoulders is acceptable.

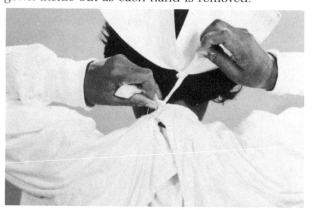

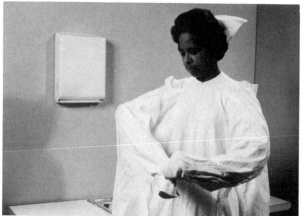

Key Steps

Touching only the inside of the gown, fold it up inside out and place it in linen bag inside the room.

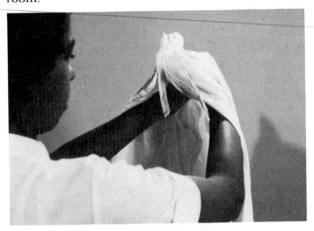

Hold gown far away from yourself while folding to avoid brushing against uniform.

Wash hands and arms well.

Turn faucet off with the paper towel used to dry hands, and use a clean towel to open door. Discard this towel outside of room.

Discussion

If gown is paper, discard it in trash receptacle. Remember that each gown is to be used only once.

Procedure for Transporting Isolated Persons

Whenever a person on isolation must leave his room for tests, isolation procedures must be continued. A person who is in respiratory isolation will only require a mask outside the room. A more stringent procedure must be followed when isolation is enteric, wound and skin, strict, or protective. Notify the department to which you are taking the person. Specify the isolation needs that will be required once you arrive.

Key Steps

Prior to entering the isolation room, drape a clean sheet over the wheelchair or stretcher.

After entering room and assisting person to stretcher or wheelchair, wrap his body with the clean sheet. Include entire body, except the head.

When returning person to his room, rewrap in sheet. After person is in room and assisted out of wheelchair or stretcher, dispose of sheet and mask inside of room.

Discussion

This will protect the stretcher or wheelchair from contamination. Protects persons on protective isolation from microorganisms.

If person is on strict isolation, also assist him to put on a mask. Sterile linen may be necessary for some persons in protective isolation (*e.g.*, burn patients).

When handling the wrap sheet, be careful not to brush it against your clothing. Wash hands well before leaving room.

Procedure for Double-Bagging Contaminated Articles

The articles that must be specially handled are those that have come in direct contact with a person who has a communicable disease and is isolated. Such items include linen, trash, and nondisposable utensils or instruments. Policies regarding this procedure may vary with each agency. Be sure you are gowned, gloved, and masked to prevent contamination.

Key Steps

Close the bag of linen or trash securely with a tight knot. This is done by a nurse standing inside of the room.

A nurse who is standing outside of the room holds a large plastic bag cuffed at the top. Hands should be covered by the cuff. The nurse inside the room gently places the contaminated bag into the clean bag, taking care not to touch the clean bag or the other nurse.

Discussion

This should be done as often as necessary. Set up a clean bag for oncoming staff.

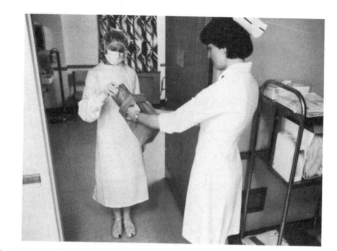

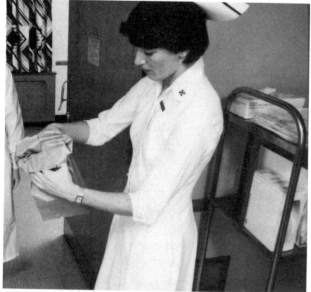

The person holding the clean bag should unroll the cuff, expel air from bag away from the face, and close securely with a knot. Then mark bag "ISOLATION" with a sticker or tape.

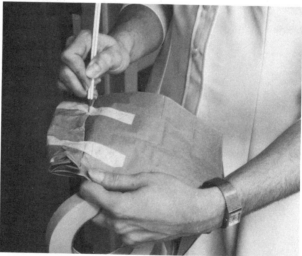

This procedure will protect personnel by double-sealing the contaminated contents and by labeling properly.

Key Steps

If removing a specimen from an isolation room, label the specimen container before entering room. Then with the same two-person approach used for linens or trash, place the labeled specimen container into a plastic bag outside the door.

Double bag contaminated equipment (*e.g.*, scissors, forceps) and remove from the room using the two-person approach.

Discussion

On laboratory slip include the type of isolation. Small, clear bags are recommended for specimens. They minimize the chance of spillage and give laboratory personnel a clear view of the specimen.

Surgical Asepsis

Surgical asepsis, or sterile technique, refers to those practices that keep surfaces void of all microorganisms. Medical asepsis, on the other hand, is intended to reduce pathogens (organisms known to cause disease). Surgical asepsis is used when the normal skin barrier is broken or a normally sterile body cavity is entered. Examples of the former include injection of medications and intravenous fluids, actual surgery, dressing changes, and wound irrigation. Examples of the latter include catheterization and tracheal suction. Surgical asepsis is also used in delivery rooms, for invasive diagnostic tests such as cardiac catheterization, in neonatal intensive care units, and for persons with decreased resistance to infection from various causes, including extensive burns, immunosuppressive drugs, leukemia, and radiation. Additional nursing procedures requiring surgical asepsis include donning of sterile gloves and gowns.

Surgical asepsis requires a sterilization procedure for all inanimate objects in order to destroy all microorganisms, including spores. There are many kinds of sterilization that use physical methods to destroy organisms. The most common of these involve the use of heat over time. Although theoretically no method kills all organisms, the practical definition of sterilization allows that only negligible organisms remain if sufficient sterilization time is used for the method and type of surface area involved. As an extra precaution to avoid possible cross contamination between patients, surgical asepsis is preferred to medical asepsis in those situations in which it is practical to sterilize rather than merely to disinfect, which is a less stringent form of organism control.

The science of microbiology underlies the principles of sterile technique, which is used in various circumstances. Regardless of the specific procedures involved, the same principles are to be followed:

- Equipment and inanimate objects that come in contact with broken skin or usually sterile body cavities are sterilized.

- When the sterility of anything is questionable, consider it unsterile.

- Sterile objects or sterile fields touch only another sterile object or surface.

- The edge of anything that encloses sterile contents is not considered sterile.

- A wet sterile surface is always considered contaminated when the surface directly under it is not sterile.
- An uncovered sterile field that is untended or out of sight is considered contaminated.
- Horizontal surfaces are considered sterile only at table level; gowns, gloves, and instruments are considered sterile only above the waistline.

Even with the best of surgical techniques, perfect asepsis is an ideal, not an absolute. Because skin cannot be sterilized, it is a common potential source of contamination in sterile procedures. Similarly, the respiratory tract cannot be rendered germ free and harbors many bacteria. Therefore, talking, coughing, or sneezing over a sterile field is to be avoided. Masks are effective only if properly used and discarded when contaminated. Gloves must be discarded when torn or contaminated. Breaks in technique must be corrected immediately, and each person is responsible for monitoring his own technique and recognizing and correcting breaks in technique. Developing a surgical conscience requires careful self-monitoring. The following list of questions may assist you to begin such a process:

1 Did you wash your hands before beginning?

2 Did you always keep your sterile field within your range of vision?

3 Did your sterile objects or sterile field touch only another sterile object or surface?

4 Did you reach around, not over, your sterile field?

5 Did you remember that 1 inch around the edge of the sterile field is considered contaminated?

6 Did your sterile field remain dry?

7 Did you cover your sterile field when it was not in use?

8 Did you keep your sterile gloved hands or sterile forceps above your waistline?

Sterile Gloves

Objective

The student will be able to do the following:

1 Don sterile gloves using principles of sterile technique.

Procedure for Donning Sterile Gloves

Key Steps

Place sealed package of sterile gloves on table or countertop.

Open the package. Touch only the outside of wrapper; open inside folder, touching only the folded edge.

Discussion

Check that package is intact and current, if dated.

Key Steps   **Discussion**

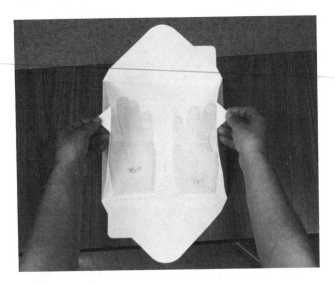

Pick up the right glove with your left hand at the fold of the cuff and pull it onto your right hand.

Touch only the inside surface of cuff.

With your gloved hand grasp the left glove under the cuff and pull it onto the left hand.

Do not allow outside glove surfaces to touch anything unsterile.

Turn up cuffs.

Touch gloved hand *only* to *outside* of other glove.

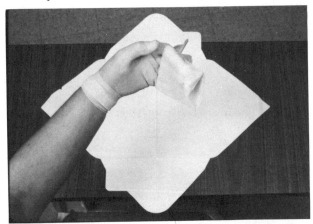

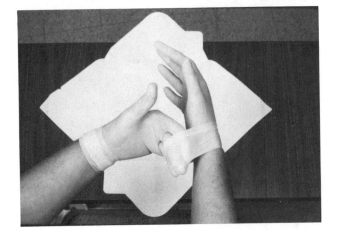

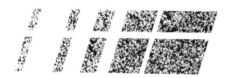

Skin

The skin is the largest organ of the body and certainly the most visible. Because the condition of the skin determines our physical appearance and attractiveness, skin alterations affect psychological as well as physiological functioning. Nurses are sensitive to both of these implications while giving care that involves the skin.

Dependent persons often require help with their skin hygiene. Again, the nurse promotes both physical and emotional well-being by assisting with this need. Providing hygiene is often a demonstration of the nurse's caring attitude.

This section includes a description of the procedures for bedbaths, dressing changes, and applications of heat and cold. Although the nurse may provide such care for the client while he is unable to care for himself, many individuals will eventually assume responsibility for these procedures. Those who will be performing their own dressing changes or applications of heat or cold at home need opportunities to practice these skills with the support of their nurse. Thus, teaching the client to participate in his own care is an important nursing responsibility.

Bedbath

Objectives

The student will be able to do the following:

1 Provide basic hygiene to a person who is unable to clean himself.
2 Provide comfort measures during the bedbath experience.
3 Demonstrate caring through verbal and nonverbal communication.
4 Assess for abilities as appropriate.

Introduction

The bedbath provides comfort and cleanliness to the person who is confined to bed and unable to perform bathing as a self-care activity. Bathing helps to remove perspiration and secretions, as well as microorganisms and sloughed skin cells. This decreases pathogens and helps to maintain an intact healthy skin. In addition to assisting with cleanliness, the bedbath provides many other opportunities as follows:

- The nurse can demonstrate a caring attitude through verbal and nonverbal communication.
- The skin can be assessed, along with peripheral vascular circulation, range of motion, and muscle tone.
- The friction of bathing can stimulate both local and systemic blood flow.
- The position changes that the person undergoes while being bathed can improve respiratory function.
- Functional abilities such as mental or phychological status may be assessed.
- Rest and relaxation may be evaluated and enhanced.
- Learning needs may be identified and teaching provided.

- The basic needs of safety and security may be met, and higher needs of self-esteem and love and belonging may also be addressed.
- A clean and comfortable appearance may enhance the person's self-esteem.

Providing personal care is an intimate experience that requires careful attention to maintain privacy and avoid unnecessary body exposure. Both exposure and evaporation of water on the skin can cause chilling, which may not only be uncomfortable but also stressful to the body in some situations.

The sensitive nurse will use the bath time to encourage advances in self-care as a means to independence and control, to the extent that the person's condition permits.

Procedure for Bedbath

Key Steps

Wash your hands.

Explain to person what you plan to do.

Answer any questions.

Bring necessary articles for hygiene and bedmaking and arrange in order of use as follows:

- Basin with warm water and soap
- Laundry bag or hamper
- Clean linen for bed
- Towel, washcloth, bath blanket (as necessary)
- Clean gown
- Other articles (*e.g.*, deodorant, toothbrush, toothpaste, razor, comb, and so forth) are usually provided by person, but the nurse should verify them.

Raise bed to comfortable working level, unless there are restrictions.

Loosen the top linen tucked under mattress. Fold spread and blanket in quarters and drape over back of chair if they are to be reused. If not, place in laundry hamper.

Discussion

Decreases anxiety.

Decreases anxiety.

An organized approach will enhance person's security, comfort, and safety.
Saves time and energy.
 Water temperature of 105° to 110°F.

Prevents strain on nurse's back.

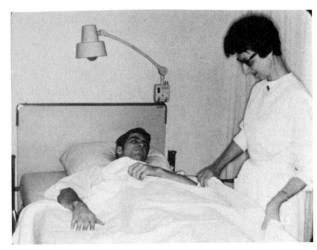

Key Steps

Keep linen away from uniform.

Place bath blanket over top sheet and remove sheet from under blanket.

Move person to side of bed in supine position to decrease need for reaching, unless it is contraindicated.

Remove gown under bath blanket.

Place towel over top part of bath blanket.

Make a mitt out of washcloth as follows:

- Tuck one edge of the washcloth under your thumb; wrap the washcloth around your hand, tucking the other edge under your thumb also.
- Bring the far edge of the washcloth over the fingers and tuck it under the near edge, in the palm of the hand. This will prevent the loose ends of the washcloth from dragging over the skin.

Discussion

Helps prevent spread of microorganisms.

Provides for privacy and also keeps patient warm. Place sheet in hamper.

Prevents unnecessary stretching and twisting by nurse.

Prevents exposure and chilling.

Towel is draped over or placed under body parts during the bath.

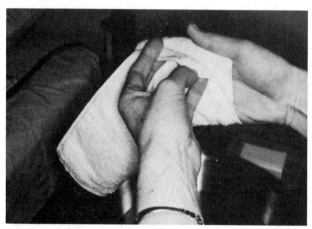

Wash person's face, often done without soap; ask person first. Also, ask if person prefers washing his own face. If he answers no, do the following:

- Wash eyes gently from the inner canthus to the outer canthus; rinse after washing each eye.
- Use firmer strokes when washing face.

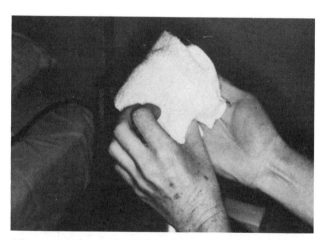

Many people prefer doing their own face washing—it is usually more comfortable.

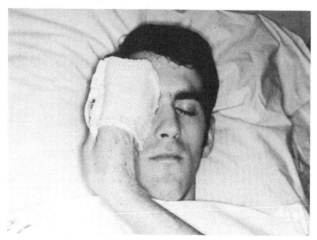

Key Steps

Discussion

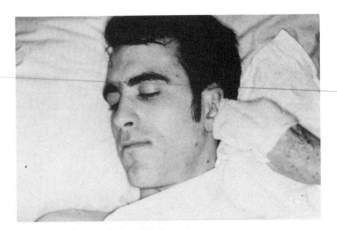

- Wash the ears well, including behind the ears. Dry face and ears well.
- Wash front and sides of neck, usually using soap. Some people bring their own soap, especially if they are allergic to certain brands. The back of the neck is more easily washed when the back is done.
- Rinse the neck and dry thoroughly.

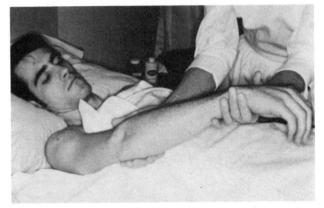

Place towel under arm farthest from you.

Wash the far hand, arm, and axilla using long, firm strokes on the arm.

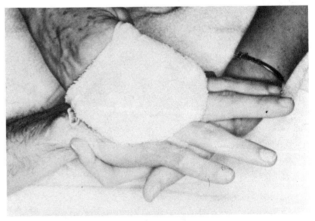

Rinse and dry thoroughly, especially between the fingers.

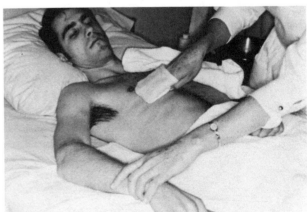

Place towel under the near arm; wash the hand, arm, and axilla in the same way.

Place towel over chest; fold bath blanket to the waist. Raise the towel with one hand, wash the chest with the other. Leave chest covered while rinsing washcloth. Rinse and dry chest. Wash, rinse, and dry thoroughly under the breasts of women.

Key Steps

Fold bath blanket down to the pubic area and leave towel over the chest to keep the person warm and to maintain privacy.

Wash, rinse, and dry lower abdomen, including the umbilicus. Remove towel, and replace bath blanket over chest and arms.

Discussion

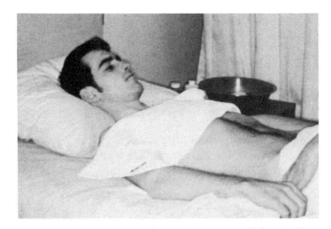

Remove bath blanket from the far leg, tucking it under the near leg and around the hip area to avoid exposure and draft.

Place towel lengthwise under the far leg.

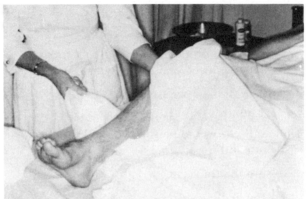

Bend the far leg at the knee. Place basin on the bed and carefully put the person's foot in the basin, so that no water is spilled. Wash the leg with long strokes; rinse and dry.

Wash and rinse the foot.

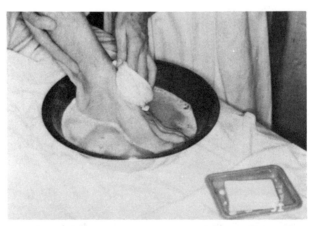

Remove basin and dry the foot well, especially between the toes.

Wash the other leg and foot in the same manner.

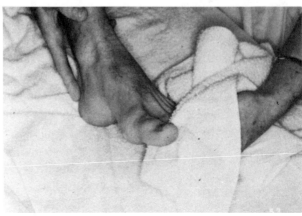

Key Steps	**Discussion**
Change bath water.	
Turn person on side or abdomen, facing away from you with the back exposed.	
Wash, rinse, and dry back and buttocks. (A backrub is sometimes given at this point or when the bath is completed.)	
Washing of the genital area is usually done by the person. The nurse often assists (*e.g.,* preparing and rinsing the washcloth).	When no assistance is needed, the nurse should pull the curtain to give privacy.
If the person is unable to do any of his private bath, the nurse should do it, washing gently from front to back, then rinsing and drying in the same direction.	
Assist the person, as necessary, with combing and arranging hair, putting on clean gown, and so forth. Men may need assistance with shaving.	Improving appearance usually contributes to boosting person's morale.
Make the occupied bed (see pp 11–13).	
Leave room in order—empty the bath basin, and clean and return it to person's room. Leave clean washcloth and towel.	
Make sure the things needed are within reach.	
Adjust the bed to person's preference, unless contraindicated.	Keeps person in alignment.

Modifications

Although bedbaths are often given daily, the frequency may be modified depending on the person's age, need, and preference. For the older person whose skin is very dry, plain water or bath lotion may be used. A modified or abbreviated bedbath may be given. This involves washing only certain parts of the body that may cause odor or discomfort if ignored daily. These include the axillae, perineal area, and back. Similarly, early A.M. care and P.M. care are hygiene measures appropriate for many persons confined to bed.

Early A.M. Care

This routine is usually performed early each morning before the activities of the day begin and before breakfast is served.

1 Offer the bedpan or urinal.
2 Pull overbed tray across the bed.
3 Supply a basin of warm water, soap, washcloth, and towel.
4 Permit the person to wash his face and hands and get ready for breakfast.
5 Give oral hygiene. (Complete this for the person if he is unable. Replace the person's dentures after rinsing them, in cold water.)
6 Straighten bed linen and fluff pillow.
7 Position bed in Fowler's position for breakfast (check Kardex first).

8 Remove wash basin and supplies, clean them, and return to storage.

P.M. Care

This routine is performed at bedtime.

1 Offer bedpan or urinal. Help person wash hands after use.

2 Assist as necessary with oral hygiene. (If person has dentures, remove them and place in denture cup; cover dentures with water, cover cup, and place in drawer of bedside stand.)

3 Provide basin of warm water, soap, washcloth, and towel; help person to wash face and hands (assist as necessary).

4 Wash and dry back; give a backrub.

5 Position person comfortably.

6 Remove, clean, and return supplies.

7 Place call bell within reach.

8 Straighten bed linens and fluff pillow.

9 Position bed to low and put side rails up.

Dressings and Wound Irrigations

Objectives

The student will be able to do the following:

1 Set up a sterile field.

2 Change a surgical dressing using sterile technique.

3 Irrigate and pack an open wound using sterile technique.

Introduction

A wound is an injury to soft tissue caused by trauma, either accidental or from surgical therapy. Because the skin is the first line of defense against microorganisms, any person with a wound where the skin surface is broken is susceptible to infection. The primary objective of nursing care for such individuals is the prevention of wound infection.

Wound Healing

Following an injury, hemorrhage and then clotting occur. Inflammation begins, and white cells initiate phagocytosis of cell debris, bacteria, and foreign matter in the wound. Fibrinogen molecules begin the formation of a fibrin network, which unites the wound edges. Fibroblasts and epithelial cells multiply, collagen proliferates, and capillary buds appear. New connective tissue is called *granulation tissue;* it is translucent, red, friable, and bleeds easily. Eventually, collagen fibers regroup to form dense scar tissue. This scar tissue contracts over a period of weeks or months until the scar becomes strong.

Healing by first intention occurs when wound edges are well approximated and no infection is present. Most surgical wounds heal by this method.

Healing by second intention occurs in large, gaping wounds that are infected. The wound is left open to drain, necrotic tissue is removed, and the wound heals by filling with granulation tissue.

Healing by third intention occurs when wound closure fails and the wound is resutured, or when a wound that is healing by second intention is closed with sutures (Fig. II-1).

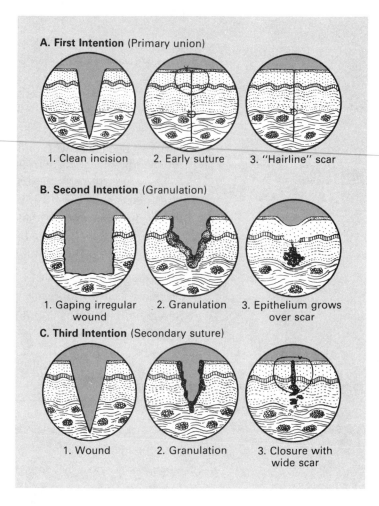

A. First Intention (Primary union)

1. Clean incision 2. Early suture 3. "Hairline" scar

B. Second Intention (Granulation)

1. Gaping irregular wound 2. Granulation 3. Epithelium grows over scar

C. Third Intention (Secondary suture)

1. Wound 2. Granulation 3. Closure with wide scar

Figure II-1

Chronologic course of wound healing by first, second, and third intention. In the final stage of second-intention healing it is to be noted that the underside of the epithelium is smooth and not serrated as normally. In the healing by second intention, the important role of contraction, which occurs in the patient in 3 dimensions and in the illustrations in 2 (B-2 and B-3), is shown. Contraction also plays a role in third-intention healing (C-2 and C-3). In C-3 an early phase is shown. Later the granulation tissue will be incorporated as a wide fibrous scar.

Dressings

Dressings may be applied to open wounds and may serve several purposes as follows:

- Mechanical barrier against microorganisms
- Protection from physical trauma
- Hemostasis, such as with tightly applied pressure dressings
- Support of underlying tissue
- Absorption of wound drainage

There are several types of dressing materials available that have different purposes. Some commonly used dressing materials include the following:

- Fine mesh gauze: closely woven material used for packing open wounds; close weave prevents new epithelial tissue from being removed with dressing.

- 4 × 4's: name refers to size; used to cover small wounds and absorb drainage from draining wounds.
- 8 × 10 abdominal pads (ABDs): large, thick, absorbent dressings; absorb drainage and provide coverage for large, draining wounds.
- Kerlix: loosely woven material that comes in rolls; useful for bandaging extremities.

Two procedures that are commonly used for treating persons with open wounds and for assisting them to attain skin integrity are described below.

Dressing Change

Superficial wounds or those that heal by first intention are often left open to the air. It is felt that undressed wounds are less likely to become infected because conditions that favor bacterial growth, such as moisture, darkness, and warmth, are avoided. However dressings may be applied to protect a wound or to absorb drainage. It is important to change dressings often enough to allow inspection of the wound's appearance. Wet dressings should be changed promptly because they act like wicks, drawing microorganisms from the environment into the wound.

Procedure for Changing a Dressing

Key Steps

Explain procedure to the person.

Wash your hands.

Collect the following equipment:

- Dressings
- Tape or Montgomery straps
- Paper or plastic bag
- Sterile gloves
- Clean gloves or disposable forceps

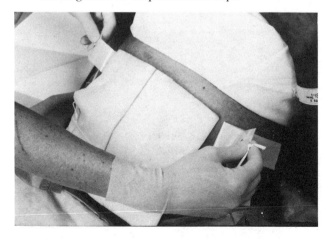

Discussion

Decreases anxiety; increases sense of control.

Decreases potential for contamination of wound.

Montgomery straps are adhesive strips with an eyelet in one end. They are applied on both sides of the wound, and gauze is threaded through the eyelets and tied to hold the dressing in place. When the dressing is changed, Montgomery straps are simply untied. Because they are left in place, they minimize trauma to the skin.

Key Steps   **Discussion**

If cleansing wound, also collect the following:

- 4 × 4's

- Antiseptic solution (as ordered by physician)

- Sterile basin

Drape person.   Provides privacy.

Open dressings and leave exposed on their sterile   Forms a sterile field.
wrappers.

OR

Open sterile towel, handling only by corners and
drape on flat surface. Open dressings and drop
onto sterile towel.

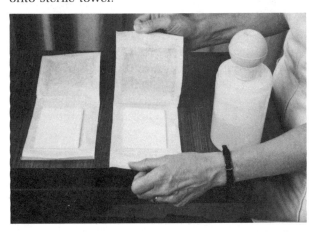

If cleansing wound do the following:
Open sterile basin; open package of 4 × 4's and
drop into basin. Pour small amount of antiseptic
solution over 4 × 4's.

Peel back tape from old dressing, pulling toward   Prevents damage to newly formed tissue.
wound.

Remove soiled dressing using clean gloves or for-   Gloves or forceps prevent spread of microorgan-
ceps. Note amount, type, and odor of drainage on   isms by way of the hands. Wound assessment per-
dressing. Note wound appearance.   mits evaluation of healing or complications.

Dispose of dressings and gloves or forceps in pa-   Controls spread of microorganisms.
per bag.

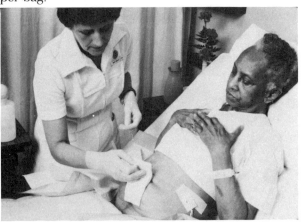

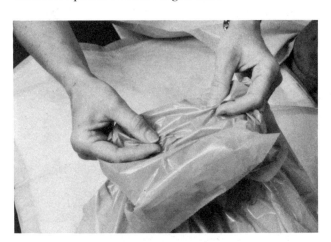

Key Steps

Discussion

Don sterile gloves.

Cleanse wound (if ordered) with moistened 4 × 4. Work from center of wound toward edges.

Prevents contaminating wound with bacteria from skin surface.

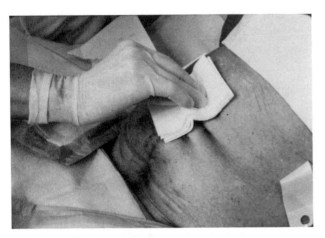

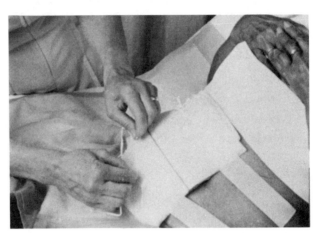

Place sterile dressings over wound.

Remove gloves.

Apply tape or Montgomery straps. Montgomery straps are left in place during dressing changes, minimizing trauma to skin.

Dispose of soiled equipment.

Chart the time of dressing change, wound appearance, and amount and type of drainage.

Wound Irrigation and Packing

Occasionally following accidental trauma or surgery, the skin and subcutaneous layers become infected. When this happens, the physician removes any skin sutures and allows the wound to open down to the fascia layer covering the muscle. This permits the infection to drain and allows the nurse and physician to debride the area. An infected wound is packed with gauze to prevent the skin from closing until the subcutaneous layers have a chance to fill in with granulation tissue. This process is known as *healing by second intention.*

Debridement of necrotic tissue can be accomplished in three ways, two of which the nurse can do with a physician's order: (1) the necrotic tissue adheres to the gauze and is pulled away when the nurse changes the dressing, and (2) the nurse irrigates the wound with solutions, such as hydrogen peroxide, that gently remove the debris. The third method of debridement, which is done by the physician, consists of dissecting the necrotic tissue from the wound.

There are few nerve endings in the subcutaneous tissue; therefore, after the first few days of irrigation, little pain is experienced. However, pain medicatons will be needed prior to irrigation for the first few days and when the physician dissects the necrotic tissue.

Procedure for Irrigating a Wound

Key Steps

Discussion

Explain procedure to the person. Implement pain-control measures.

Decreases anxiety.
Relaxation techniques or pain medication may be needed for comfort.

Wash your hands.

Collect the following equipment:

- Wound irrigation set
- Dressings
- Sterile solution for irrigation as ordered by physician
- Blue pad(s)
- Tape or Montgomery straps
- Paper or plastic bag
- Sterile gloves
- Clean gloves or plastic disposable forceps

When you open a new bottle of solution, the *date* and *time* must be written on the label. Solutions are not considered sterile after they have been open for 24 hours. Discard any solution left in the bottle.
When pouring solutions, have the label face you—pour away from yourself (*e.g.*, place palm of hand over label when grasping bottle, and direct fluid stream away from yourself).

Prepare the sterile field as follows:

- Open irrigation set
- Place dressing material on sterile field

Dressing materials should be placed on the sterile field so that they are in the order in which they will be used (*e.g.*, 8 × 10's on bottom, 4 × 4's next, and fine mesh gauze on the top).

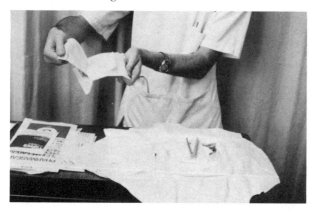

Drape person.

Place blue pad under person.

Place plastic or paper bag so tht you can reach it easily.

Provides privacy.

Catches any spilled fluid.

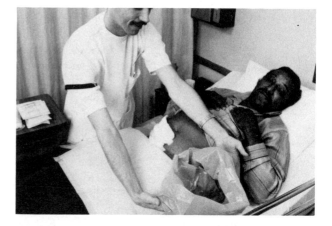

Key Steps	Discussion

Key Steps

Remove soiled dressings with clean gloves or plastic disposable forceps.

Note amount, type, and odor of drainage.
Note wound appearance.

Drop soiled dressings in the paper or plastic bag.

Assist person into comfortable position, which will also allow for maximum drainage.

Loosen bottle cap(s) on irrigation solution(s).

Put on *one* sterile glove. Use this hand to remove irrigation container from sterile basin, and place level on sterile field. Remove bulb syringe from container.

Use *unsterile* hand to remove bottle cap. Set cap on level surface with inside facing up.

Continue to use unsterile hand to pour solution(s) into container. Use measurement markings on container to measure approximte amounts of solution.

Return cap(s) to solution bottle(s).

Put on the other *sterile* glove. Remove the cap from the end of the bulb syringe and place syringe in irrigation container.

Place sterile basin near the wound.

Irrigate wound until all solution has been used and the majority of fluid has drained out of the wound. The solution washes away microorganisms, tissue debris, and drainage.

Discussion

Avoid touching the soiled dressings with your hands to both keep from spreading microorganisms from your hands onto the wound and to prevent the spread of microorganisms from the wound to yourself and others.

Wound assessment allows evaluation of progress of wound healing.

Gravity causes liquids to flow from high to lower levels.

This facilitates pouring solution(s) and maintaining sterile equipment and sterile field simultaneously.

Maintains sterility of the inside of the cap.

Decreases exposure of bottle contents to airborne microorganisms.

The basin should be placed below the level of the wound to catch the drainage. The person can hold the basin, but if he does handle the basin, it is unsterile and you cannot touch it until the procedure is complete. When handing the basin to the person, do not let him touch your gloves.

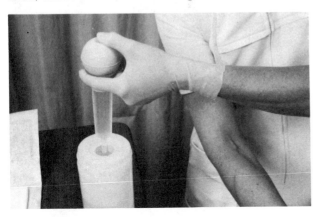

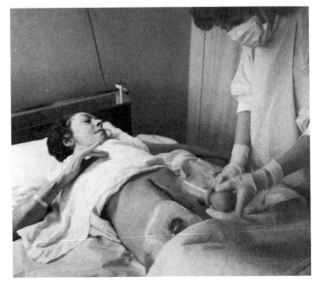

Key Steps   **Discussion**

Pack the wound as follows:

- Line with gauze (open to full size).

~~The wound is lined so that all of the packing can~~
be removed later by pulling out the lining rather
than picking out each individual piece

- Take gauze, unfold it completely, wrinkle it
  into a ball (a fluff), and place it into the wound.

- Use as many fluffs as necessary to fill the   Be sure to fully pack the corners of the wound
  wound.   to prevent abscesses from forming.

Place 4 × 4's over wound to absorb any drainage
that cannot be fully absorbed by the gauze
packing.

Put on 5 × 9's, 8 × 10's or ABDs to absorb drainage and hold packing and 4 × 4's in place.

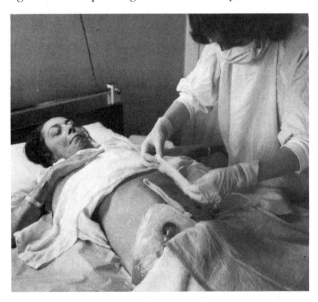

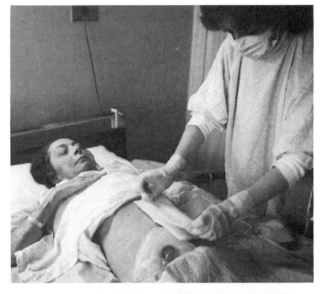

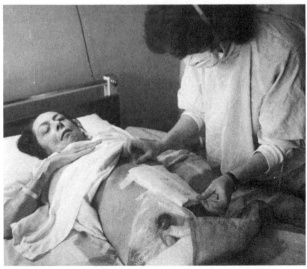

Remove gloves and discard.

Secure dressing in place with tape or Montgomery
straps. Because Montgomery straps do not require
changing with each dressing change, they are used
on dressings that need to be changed frequently in
order to minimize trauma to skin.

Assist person to comfortable position.

Discard used materials.

Chart the time of procedure, wound appearance,
and amount and type of wound drainage.

Application of Heat and Cold

Objectives

The student will be able to do the following:

1 Describe purposes of hot and cold applications.

2 Discuss principles of conduction and convection in relation to heat and cold therapy.

3 Implement dry and moist heat and cold therapies safely.

Introduction

People require narrow ranges of environmental and body temperature for survival. However, both heat and cold can also be used to help adapt to altered body function. Specifically, heat or cold applied to the body can change temperature locally or systemically for a therapeutic purpose. Both heat and cold may be used as dry or moist applications. Body response to heat and cold is determined by the manner, intensity, and duration of application, the nature and condition of underlying tissue, and the amount of body surface covered by the application.

The principles of conduction and radiation apply to both intentional application of heat and cold for therapeutic purposes and potential misuse of heat and cold.

In conduction heat passes directly from molecule to molecule. The following are examples:

- Hot wet compresses (moist heat)
- Heating pad (dry heat)
- Cold wet compresses (moist cold)
- Ice bag (dry cold)

In radiation heat transfers from warmer to cooler objects by electromagnetic rays. One example is a heat lamp (dry heat).

Heat applications are used to increase the following:

- Vasodilation
- Metabolism
- Circulation
- Temperature
- Suppuration (pus formation)

and to decrease the following:

- Pain
- Muscle tension
- Viscosity of exudate

Cold applications are used to increase the following:

- Vasoconstriction
- Local anesthesia

and to decrease the following:

- Inflammation
- Temperature
- Metabolism

The principles of sterile technique may be required in either the application of heat or cold. Extended exposure to both heat and cold can cause severe tissue damage. Essentially, the time, distance, and shielding from the source of heat or cold are important considerations in assuring the safe application of both.

Procedure for Applying Dry Heat

Key Steps

Gather the following equipment:

- Heating device
- Towel or other covering
- Tape or ties (as needed)

Explain procedure. Inform person that heat application will feel warm, not hot.

Assess the person's skin.

Prepare heat source and wrap in cloth cover, such as a towel.

Hot water bottles:

- Fill hot water bottles ½ to ⅔ full with water at 115°F (46°C).
- Press remaining air out of bag and close bag.

Heating pads:

- Should be set no higher than "low" to prevent burns.
- Most pads come with their own covering.

Aqua (K) pads:

- Prepare by adding distilled water to the control unit and plugging unit into electrical outlet.
- The temperature setting is adjustable only with a plastic key.

Discussion

Some methods of direct application of dry heat are the following:

- Hot water bottle—rarely used in institutions because of danger of burns.
- Electric heating pads—used less often than in the past in institutions because of danger of burns when set on "high." Commonly used in homes.
- Aqua (K) pads—similar to a heating pad, but heat is provided by warm water circulated by a motorized control unit rather than electric wires.
- Commercially prepared packs—contain chemicals that react to provide heat when activated.

Facilitates client participation in safe use of device. Burns can occur when clients increase the temperature of the heat source, expecting applications to feel hot.

Heat is not applied to areas of erythema and blisters. Likewise, heat should not be applied to areas where circulation is impaired (e.g., lower extremities in persons with vascular occlusive disease), because heat increases metabolic demands of tissues, which cannot be met by impaired blood supply.

Cloth covers prevent possible burns from direct contact with heat source.

Key Steps	*Discussion*
• Free rubber hoses from kinks to allow water to circulate freely, and turn switch to "on."	
Commercially prepared packs:	
• Squeeze or deliver sharp blow to commercial packs according to package directions.	
Shield person as needed for modesty and apply heat source to dry skin.	Because water conducts heat, drying skin prevents burns.
Secure device and leave application in place for prescribed time.	Applications are usually left on 20 minutes to 30 minutes to decrease the potential for reflex vasoconstriction.
Assess person during and after heat application for signs of thermal injury, such as pain, erythema, or blistering. Assess for therapeutic effects (*e.g.*, decreased pain or inflammation).	Prevents possible tissue damage, and evaluates effectiveness of therapy.
Chart the time, duration, and type of treatment, and person's response.	Provides documentation.

Procedure for Application of Dry Cold

Key Steps	*Discussion*
Gather the following equipment: • Cold appliance • Protective covering • Tape or ties (as needed)	Some methods of applying dry cold are the following: • Ice bag—rubber bag that is filled with crushed ice. • Ice collar—an elongated bag that is applied to the neck. • Commercially prepared cold pack—contain chemicals that react to produce cold when activated.
Explain procedure.	Enables client to participate safely in care. Ask him to inform you if pain or burning sensation occurs during treatment.
Assess skin condition.	Note signs of impaired circulation or areas of diminished sensation. Cold application to those areas may cause tissue damage.
Prepare cold source.	Fill ice bags ½ to ⅔ full with crushed ice, press out remaining air and close bag. Squeeze or deliver sharp blow to commercial packs according to package directions.
Cover device with cloth.	Absorbs condensation that collects on device, and protects skin from possible injury from direct application.
Shield person as needed for privacy and modesty. Apply and secure device.	

Key Steps	**Discussion**
Leave in place for the prescribed time.	Time is usually 30 minutes or less to decrease potential for reflex vasodilation.
Assess for signs of injury during and after treatment, such as erythema, pallor, cyanosis, numbness, burning, or pain. Assess for therapeutic effects (e.g., decreased pain, swelling, or bleeding).	Prevents tissue injury, and evaluates effectiveness of treatment.
Chart the time, duration, and type of cold application, and person's response.	Provides documentation.

Procedure for Applying Moist Compresses

Key Steps	**Discussion**
Gather the follow equipment: • Water or prescribed solution, warmed or cooled to appropriate temperature • Gauze dressings or cloth • Towel • Plastic pad or sheeting • Heating device or ice bag (if desired) • Tape or ties • Sterile gloves (for sterile application)	Solution temperature is as follows: • For hot compresses, 100°F (43°C). • For cold compresses, 59°F (15°C). Commercially prepared premoistened packs are available for hot compresses. They are heated infrared devices. Use sterile equipment if skin is not intact.
Moisten gauze or cloth with water or prescribed solution and wring until just damp.	Prevents discomfort from dripping.
Apply to affected part and cover with plastic.	Insulates compresses to maintain therapeutic temperature.
Apply heating device or ice bag (if desired) and cover pack with a towel. Secure with tape or ties.	Heating devices or ice bags are helpful for maintaining compress at a therapeutic temperature. Towel provides additional insulation.
Leave in place for prescribed length of time.	Time is usually 15 minutes to 30 minutes to decrease potential for reflex vasoconstriction or vasodilation.
Assess person for signs of thermal injury and therapeutic effects.	See pp 40 through 42 for specific observations.
Chart the time, duration, and type of compress applied, and person's response.	Provides documentation.

Other Considerations

Additional means of applying heat include heat lamps and soaks. Heat lamps provide heat by radiation from an electric bulb. They are used to dry skin areas that have become excoriated from moisture or to increase circulation in injured areas, for example, decubitus ulcers. Heat lamps are positioned 18 inches to 24 inches from the affected area, a low-watt bulb is used, and therapy usually lasts 15 minutes to 20 minutes to prevent possible burns. Be careful not to position the lamp where it can touch linens, and instruct the person not to touch the bulb to prevent fire or injury.

Soaks involve immersion of a body part in warm water (110°F or 43°C). Soaks are applied for approximately 20 minutes and are used to increase local circulation, relieve pain, or cleanse open wounds. A sitz bath is a special type of soak involving the pelvic area. The person may sit in a bathtub in water up to his waist, in a commercially available tub that is designed to fit in the toilet seat, or in a chair that is molded to hold water. Watch for fainting after sitz baths caused by blood pooling in the dilated vessels of the pelvic area.

The nurse can be helpful in providing suggestions for hot and cold applications in the home. A can of frozen juice covered with a cloth or a plastic bag filled with ice cubes make easily prepared cold packs. A popsicle can be used to apply cold for a youngster with a mouth injury. Towels soaked in hot water and enclosed in a plastic wrap are effective hot compresses. The nurse can also be an important source of information regarding the safe use of hot and cold applications and devices.

Mobility

From infancy to old age, we take for granted our ability to move about. Through body mobility, we assert personal independence while performing activities of daily living and interacting with others. Alterations in mobility may occur for a variety of reasons, including bed rest and motor restrictions imposed for other health problems, actual impairment of motor structures or process, or generalized weakness.

A careful assessment including range of motion (ROM) of various joints may be necessary to determine the extent of mobility possible. The person should be assisted to be as mobile as possible within the limits of medical restrictions, physical ability, and tolerance. As discussed in many chapters of the accompanying text, mobility affects and is affected by other biopsychosocial statuses. The basic procedures discussed here are those most often used to maintain optimal structural alignment and motor function. They include passive range of motion, positioning, and lifting and moving.

Passive Range of Motion

Objectives

The student will be able to do the following:

1 Use passive and active exercises appropriately.
2 State the complete ranges of motion for each joint.
3 Move joints within free range of motion.
4 Support extremities appropriately during range of motion.
5 Document any unexpected response to range-of-motion exercises.

Introduction

Most people normally exercise their joints when carrying out activities of daily living. When activity is limited, special measures are needed to maintain joint mobility and, in turn, physical condition. With extreme limitation of activity, muscles may contract and atrophy, and joints may become fixed. To the extent that the person is able to perform the exercises that provide range of motion, he should be encouraged to do so. He may require instruction by the nurse of specific movements to be used. There are two types of range-of-motion exercises:

- Active exercise (performed by the person)—muscle contraction is present.
- Passive exercise (motion performed by the nurse or another person for the client)—no muscle contraction occurs.

When performing the motion for the client, the nurse uses both hands and stabilizes the proximal joint (closest to trunk) and moves the distal joint (farthest from trunk). If the body of the muscle is grasped, pain and injury may occur. During passive exercise the client lies in a comfortable position in good body alignment to decrease the pull of gravity on the total body. With passive exercise, the person is totally relaxed and does not assist with exercise but notifies the nurse if he experiences discomfort. The types of motions that may be used are the following:

1 Abduction—movement away from midline of the body

2 Adduction—movement of a limb toward the center of the body

3 Extension—straightening out of the joint

4 Flexion—bending the joint

5 Hyperextension—extending a joint beyond the ordinary range

6 Pronation—turning downward

7 Supination—turning upward

Procedure for Passive Range of Motion

Key Steps

Raise bed to convenient height.

Stand on side of body part to be moved.

Put joints through normal motion as follows:

- Neck
  - Flexion
  - Extension
  - Rotation

Discussion

Minimizes strain on nurse's muscles

All movements should be gentle and rhythmic to promote comfort and express caring.

Support head; move head.

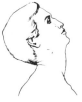

Extension neutral

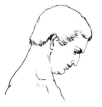

Flexion

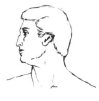

Rotation

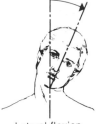

Lateral flexion

- Shoulder
  - Flexion
  - Extension
  - Abduction
  - Adduction
  - Internal rotation
  - External rotation
  - Hyperextension

Stabilize shoulder girdle; move arm.

Done in prone position.

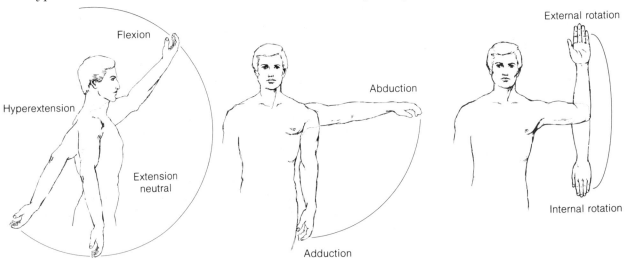

Flexion

Hyperextension

Extension neutral

Abduction

Adduction

External rotation

Internal rotation

Key Steps

Discussion

- Elbow
  Flexion
  Extension
  Supination
  Pronation

Stabilize arm; move forearm.

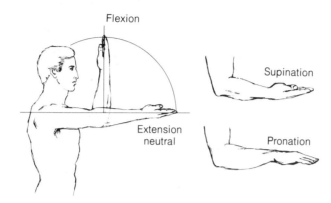

- Wrist
  Flexion (dorsi and palmar)
  Extension
  Ulnar deviation
  Radial deviation

Stabilize forearm; move hand.

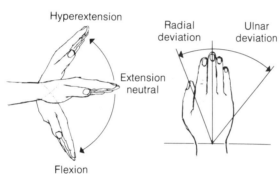

- Joints of fingers
  Metacarpophalangeal joints
  Flexion
  Extension
  Abduction
  Adduction
  Interphalangeal joints
  Flexion
  Extension

Stabilize metacarpals of hand; move fingers.

Stabilize proximal or middle phalanx; move middle and distal phalanx.

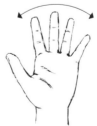

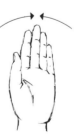

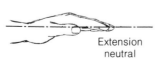

Key Steps	**Discussion**

Thumb

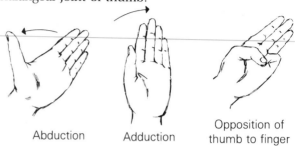

Stabilize metacarpals and wrist; move metacarpo-phalangeal joint of thumb.

Flexion
Extension
Abduction
Adduction
Opposition

Flexion

Extension neutral

Abduction   Adduction   Opposition of thumb to finger

Especially important—without full use of thumb, hand function is severely limited.

• Hip
    Flexion
    Extension
    Abduction
    Adduction
    Internal rotation
    External rotation
    Hyperextension

Stabilize pelvis; move thigh.

Done in prone position.

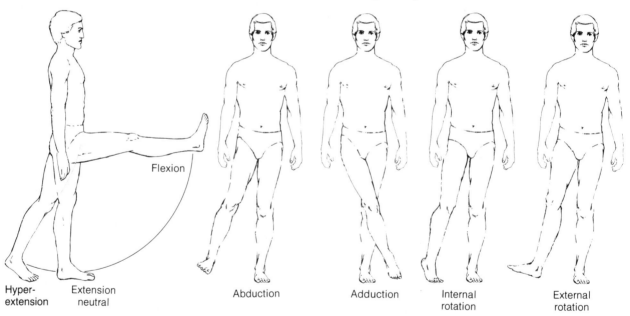

Flexion

Hyper-extension   Extension neutral   Abduction   Adduction   Internal rotation   External rotation

• Knee
    Flexion
    Extension

Extension neutral

Flexion

Stabilize thigh; move leg.

Done in prone position.

Key Steps	*Discussion*
• Ankle 　Dorsiflexion 　Plantar flexion 　　Eversion 　　Inversion	Stabilize leg; move foot.

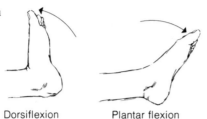 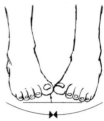 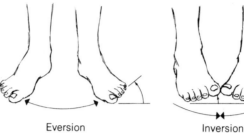

Dorsiflexion	Plantar flexion	Eversion	Inversion

• Toe 　Interphalangeal joint	Stabilize proximal or middle joint phalanx; move middle and distal phalanx.
Flexion 　　Extension 　Metacarpophalangeal joint 　　Flexion 　　Extension 　　Abduction 　　Adduction	Stabilize metatarsal; move proximal phalanx.

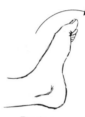 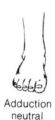

Extension neutral	Flexion	Adduction neutral	Abduction

Return all joints to neutral position.	Maintains functional alignment.
Document any unexpected response.	

Modifications

- The specific joints to exercise and the number of times to move each joint vary with the person's condition. It is more effective and less tiring to repeat a smaller number of exercises several times a day.

- Isometric exercises actively contract and relax muscles without moving joints. These exercises may be prescribed or suggested to strengthen certain muscle groups, for example, abdominal, large muscles of the thighs, or perineal muscles.

- Resistive exercises are prescribed by physicians and may be performed by physical therapists. This is active exercise carried out by a person working against resistance (mechanical or manual).

Positioning

Objectives

The student will be able to do the following:

1 Position persons to maintain correct body alignment when confined to bed.

2 Provide safety in various circumstances.

3 Provide comfort and relaxation.

4 Maintain and improve physiologic functioning.

Introduction

Positioning maintains body alignment, thereby affecting both structure and function. Changing positions stimulates specific physiological functions such as circulation, elimination, and respiration. Proper support and frequent position change facilitate relaxation and comfort by purposefully resting various muscle groups. Without proper position and support, dysfunctional alignment occurs. The effects of gravity and pull of strong flexor muscles can lead to flexion contractures, abnormal rotation of ball and socket joints (*e.g.*, external rotation), and foot drop (contracture of gastrocnemius and soleus muscles). Without frequent change of position, the dependent person is at high risk for skin breakdown or pressure sores, especially at weight-bearing bony prominences where bone is covered by skin and minimal amounts of subcutaneous fat.

The nurse provides position changes as needed. These changes will be consistent with the physician's orders and based on the nurse's clinical judgment.

The basic protective positions for the person lying in bed are the following:

- Supine (dorsal recumbent)
- Prone (face-lying)
- Semi-prone
- Side-lying
- Fowler's

Procedure for Supine (Dorsal Recumbent) Position

Key Steps

Place bed in flat position.

Position person flat in bed on back in proper alignment.

- Keep spine straight.

- Avoid neck flexion.

- Place a footboard at right angles to lower legs and position so feet are against it.

- Prevent external rotation of the femurs by positioning legs straight with toes pointed up, not out.

- Observe result of positioning.

Discussion

Requires firm support mattress or bed board to avoid exaggerated curve of spine and hip flexion.

If a head pillow is used, it should be small and placed under head, neck, and upper shoulder.

Foot drop occurs when gravity pulls feet into plantar flexion.

Use sandbags or trochanter roll.

Is body in straight line?
Are toes pointed to ceiling?
Is trochanter roll preventing leg from moving outward?

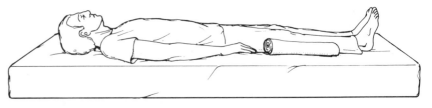

Key Steps	**Discussion**
	Ask person if he feels he could remain in this position for 1 hour to 2 hours.
Draw top sheet over footboard or bed cradle to keep pressure from toes.	A top sheet can also pull feet into plantar flexion if it is too tight over toes.
Replace call bell, and secure side rails.	

Procedure for Prone (Face-lying) Position

Key Steps	**Discussion**
Place bed in flat position.	
Position person flat on abdomen in good alignment.	
• Keep spine straight	
• Keep toes off the mattress	Place toes over bottom of mattress, or support legs on pillows to prevent foot drop and pressure on toes, which could result in skin breakdown.
• Avoid neck flexion	Place a small pillow or turn head to side directly on mattress.
• Place arms parallel to body in slightly flexed position or at side, elbows flexed to 90°.	Keeps body weight off arms, and promotes comfort.

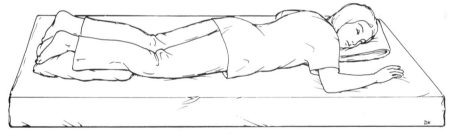

Key Steps	**Discussion**
Observe result of positioning.	
• Are head, trunk, and legs aligned?	A small pillow may be used at lower ribs and upper abdomen to ease breathing.
• Are toes pointed downward and off bed?	
• Ask person if he feels pressure on chest or genitals.	
Replace call bell, and secure side rails.	

Procedure for Semi-prone Position

Key Steps	**Discussion**
Place bed in flat position.	
Position person between prone and side-lying.	
• Place pillows to support entire trunk.	Position one or two pillows under abdomen to prevent person from slipping into prone position.

Key Steps   *Discussion*

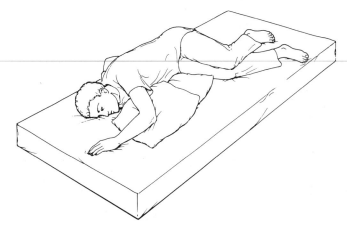

- Put person's lower arm behind him.   Keeps body weight off arm.
- Hyperextend neck slightly.   Use small pillow under head.
- Flex upper leg slightly.   May need folded bath blanket to cushion
                                                 between legs.

Observe result of position.   Is shoulder supported sufficiently to facilitate
                                                 breathing?
                                                 Ask person if he feels comfortable.

Replace call bell, and secure side rails.

Procedure for Side-lying Position

Key Steps   *Discussion*

Place bed in flat position.

Raise person's arm on side on which he is to be   This will prevent person from rolling on arm when
positioned and rest arm on head pillow.   being positioned on side.

Position person on side.
- Put pillow under head.   Counters lateral neck rotation.
- Place pillow in front of chest and put person's   Lower arm is flexed 90° at elbow and placed
  arm on it.   alongside pillow to prevent lying on arm.
- Place pillow in front of thigh and put top leg
  on it.
- Straighten lower leg.

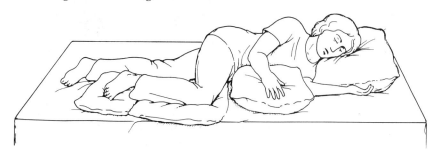

Key Steps

Observe result of position.

Replace call bell, and secure side rails.

Discussion

Are head, neck, and back aligned?
Does person look comfortable?
To avoid strain at hip or shoulder, roll supporting pillow at back or top; hip may be repositioned slightly forward.
Ask person if he feels comfortable.

Procedure for Fowler's Position

Key Steps

Place person with hips at angle of elevation.

Elevate seat of bed 15° to 20°.

Elevate foot of bed 15° to 20°.

Elevate head of bed to highest position (70° to 90°).

Place small pillow behind head and shoulders, or rest head against bed. Place pillows under arms.

Discussion

Keeps back straight.

Greater flexion or pillow at knees causes excess pressure, which compromises circulation and nerve function.

Gravity aids circulation and counteracts foot drop. If foot of bed is not elevated, use footboard.

Gravity pulls abdominal organs away from chest cavity, increasing heart and lung efficiency.

Avoids flexion of neck and pull on shoulders.

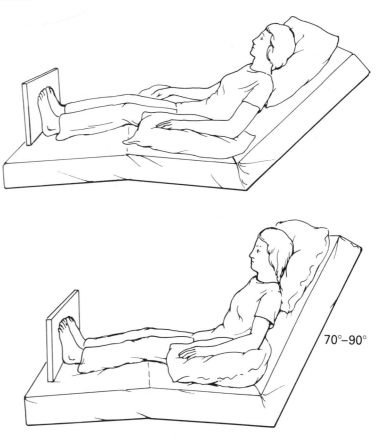

70°–90°

Key Steps	**Discussion**
Observe result of position.	Are head, trunk, and legs aligned? Is head bent too far on chest? Ask person if he feels the following: • Strain on shoulders • As if falling to one side • Strain on back If he does, turn pillow lengthwise, or a second pillow can be used.

Replace call bell, and secure side rails.

Modifications

Sometimes the head of bed (HOB) is placed at 30° to 45° for semi-Fowler's position. The semi-sitting position facilitates eating and other activities of daily living.

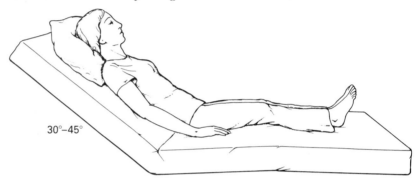

Lifting and Moving

Objectives

The student will be able to do the following:

1 State the appropriate body mechanics to use for lifting and moving activities.
2 Use appropriate methods to turn and position the person.
3 Correctly transfer a person to stretcher or chair.
4 Ambulate person appropriately.
5 Ensure safety of persons during moving and transfer.

Introduction

When a person is unable to meet mobility needs independently, the nurse assists with these functions. It is the responsibility of the nurse to maintain the safety of the person as well as his or her own personal safety during lifting and moving procedures.

   The nurse recognizes that mobility affects many other body functions, including circulation, respiration, and bowel elimination. Immobility subjects the person to increased risk of diminished strength for activities of daily living, skin breakdown, and even demineralization of bones. Additionally, those who are unable to move independently may be prone to sensory overload or sensory deprivation in their restricted environments.

   Sometimes position and movement may be prescribed by the

physician. At other times, the nurse will determine the nature and frequency of interventions that involve lifting and moving the person. Commonly used techniques are the following:

- Moving a person up in bed
- Turning a person in bed (back to side)
- Moving a person from bed to stretcher
- Assisting a person from bed to chair
- Assisting a person to ambulate

Remember, when you position or move a person, always perform the activity "with," rather than "to," the person.

Procedure for Moving a Person up in Bed

Key Steps

Lower head of bed, and remove pillow.

Assess person's ability to assist.

If person is able to assist, ask him to flex knees and push feet into bed.

Place one arm under person's shoulders, the other under his hips to support sacral area.

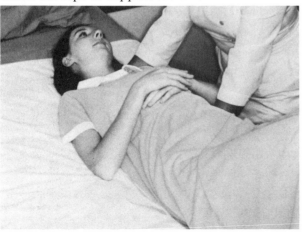

Discussion

Lifting or sliding across a flat surface requires less effort.

Having person assist encourages independence and use of muscles that aid in maintaining circulation, respiration, and mobility.

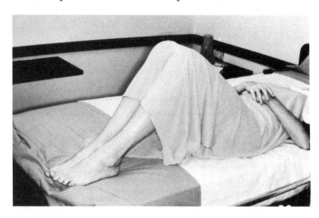

Dragging the buttocks causes tissue layers to move on each other, constricting blood supply and causing shearing force tissue damage.

Key Steps	**Discussion**
Move carefully toward head of bed on signal.	Avoids hitting head against bed.
Raise the seat and knee gatch after person is properly positioned.	Prevents sliding down in bed.
Adjust covers.	Provides for privacy.
Replace call bell and secure side rails.	Provides for safety.

Modifications and Comments

There are alternate methods for moving a person up in bed. If a person is able to assist by pushing with his legs, the locked-arm method or grasping the head of the bed while pushing with his feet are very effective. The use of a mechanical aid, such as a trapeze, is useful for persons with limited use of their legs. With a trapeze, they can use their arms to assist in pulling up in bed.

If a person is unable to assist in moving up in bed, two nurses can accomplish this by using a double locked-arm method or a drawsheet (see procedure for Moving a Person from Bed to Stretcher, p 60).

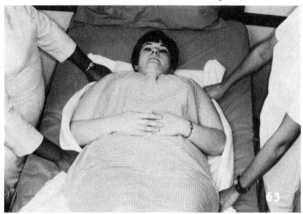 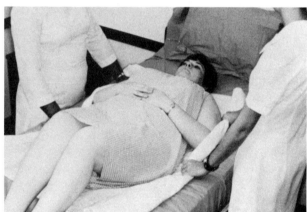

Procedure for Turning a Person in Bed (Back to Side)

Key Steps	**Discussion**
Identify person's individual need for turning and any modifications necessary.	Purposes include the following: • Promotes skin integrity and comfort. • Assists in circulation and respiration.
Assess need for assistance. Two or more nurses may be needed if person is very heavy or helpless.	Avoids possibility of strain to nurse.
Explain what is to be done and how person can help.	Decreases anxiety and encourages person's help as he is able.
Adjust bed to convenient height.	Lifting requires countering gravity. Minimizes strain on nurse's muscles.
Drop side rail, and stand at bedside using a wide stance and bent knees and hips.	Bringing weight close to body and creating a broad base assists balance.

Key Steps

Move person toward you, placing hands palm up under shoulders, hips, legs, and feet in turn.

To prevent the person from rolling onto his arm, place the near arm across the chest and other arm alongside head.

Ask person to flex knees, if able. If person is unable, cross near ankle over far ankle for same purpose.

Turn the person smoothly and avoid twisting and jarring.

Inform person you are ready to turn and then perform turn. This action provides for person to assist, if possible.

Discussion

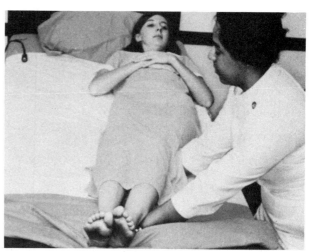

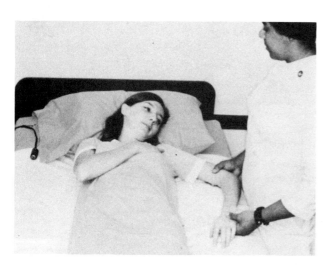

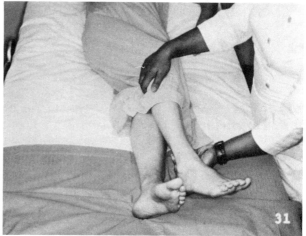

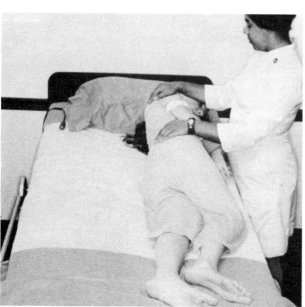

Key Steps	Discussion
Readjust alignment.	Preserves musculoskeletal integrity.
Once proper body alignment is achieved, supports may be necessary to maintain position (*e.g.*, rolled pillows at back).	Maintains position by preventing person from rolling back. Maintains alignment.
Use supports such as pillows, towels, or bath blankets between legs and ankles.	Prevents friction and skin breakdown by separating bony prominences.
Adjust covers for privacy.	
Replace call bell, and secure side rails for safety.	

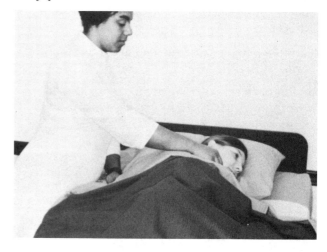

Modifications and Comments

Turning provides the opportunity for many observations, especially of skin condition. Note unusual observations, and institute appropriate interventions. In the absence of lung complications and actual skin breakdown, turning every 2 hours may be appropriate.

Procedure for Moving a Person from Bed to Stretcher

Key Steps	Discussion
If person can assist: Remove covers, and substitute bath blankets.	Provides privacy and warmth.
Raise bed height to above stretcher.	Uses gravity to advantage.
Place stretcher parallel to length of bed and even with head.	
Lock wheels of both bed and stretcher. Hold stretcher against bed with body to provide for safety.	

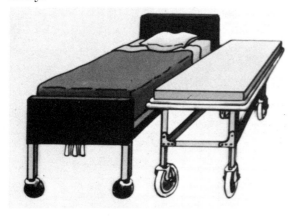

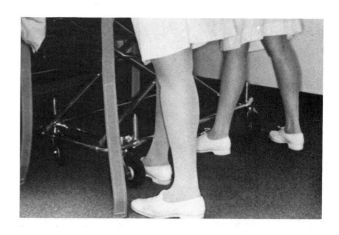

Key Steps	*Discussion*
Use one hand to support person under shoulder and other hand to grasp his far hand.	Provides leverage for person to pull toward stretcher.
Have person move hips, then shoulders, until positioned in center of stretcher.	Assists in a smooth transfer.
Place pillow under head, and position arms at side.	Provides comfort and safety.
Lift near side rail. Secure safety belt across person. Unlock stretcher wheels. Move stretcher slightly to access other side rail. Push stretcher feet first.	

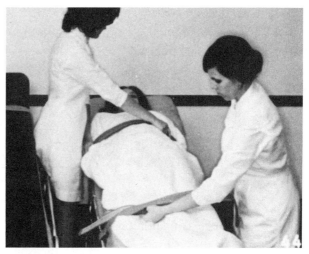

If person cannot assist (drawsheet method):
Assess size and weight of person, and obtain assistance. One to three assistants may be needed.

Maintains safety of nurse and person during transfer.

Raise bed height to above stretcher.

Uses gravity to advantage.

Place a draw sheet or pull sheet under person's buttocks and upper thighs to permit maximal lift under the heaviest body part.

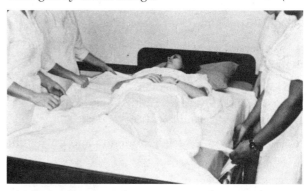

Tighten sheet into a hammock by folding or rolling it toward the person's sides.

A tight and secure sheet prevents slipping or jarring of person during transfer.

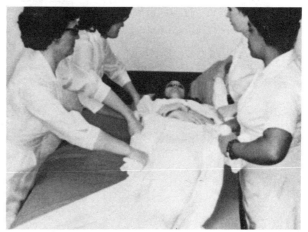

Key Steps	**Discussion**
Place stretcher parallel to length of bed and even with head.	
Lock wheels of both bed and stretcher.	
Position assistants to support chest and abdomen, and pelvis and hips.	Evenly distributes weight of person to accomplish a safe, smooth transfer.
With a very heavy person and a short nurse, the nurse may kneel on edge of bed.	Permits better leverage and body mechanics.
Lift person to stretcher in synchronized motion to provide smooth, safe transfer.	

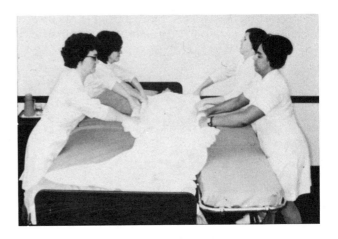

If person cannot assist (three-person carry): Obtain assistance; two additional persons are needed.

Allows lifters room to manuever.

Position stretcher at right angles to the bed, with head of stretcher nearly touching foot of bed.

Provides safety.

Lock wheels of both stretcher and bed.

Place all three lifters on same side of bed.

Place tallest lifter at head or strongest lifter at hips.

Cross person's ankle toward lifters. Place lifters' hands, palms up, under the person.

Facilitates turn.

On signal, lift simultaneously with cradled arms, drawing person up and facing lifters. Person's weight will rest against carriers' chests.

Carry person to stretcher smoothly and in rhythm.

Person will experience security and minimal jarring.

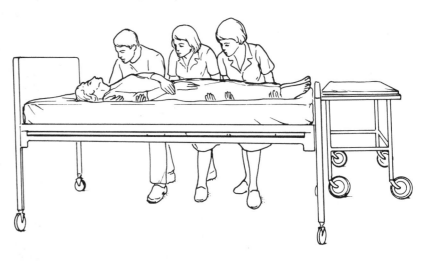

Key Steps   **Discussion**

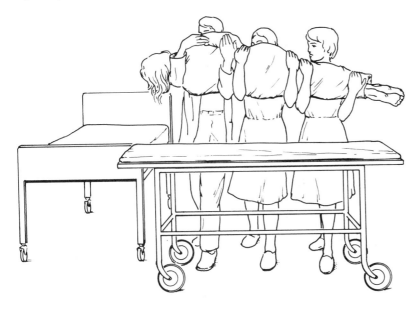

Place pillow under head and arms at side. Secure safety belt across person, and lift side rails.

Unlock stretcher wheels and push stretcher feet first.

Provides comfort and safety.

Procedure for Assisting a Person from Bed to Chair

Key Steps

Identify person's individual needs and any appropriate modifications.

Encourage person's help as he is able.

Anticipate need for privacy and for bedpan or urinal.

Place bed in lowest position.

Position chair and lock wheels of both bed and chair. Place chair parallel to foot of bed with seat facing head of bed; footrest should be turned out of way.

Discussion

Various modifications will be required for persons with left or right hemiplegia or casts.

Person may have preferences.

Screen person carefully, and wash hands appropriately.

Ensures safety.

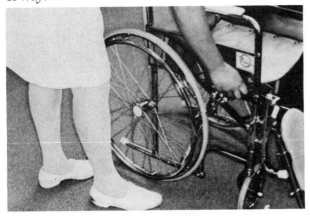

Key Steps

Assist person to sitting position in bed.

Observe person for tolerance before proceeding.

Assist person to dangle legs over side of bed.

Assist person to standing position.
- Nurse places one leg between person's legs, one to outside.
- Person places hands on nurse's shoulders.

Discussion

Raise head of bed. Stand facing person and offer support using locked-arm method or support of shoulders. Remember to maintain straight back and use large muscles of arms and legs.

Nurse may need to support shoulders and lift legs over edge. Dangling allows circulatory adaptation. Monitor pulse.

Nurse's stance provides balance and wide base of support. Ask person to raise body as you lift, using bent hips and knees.
Place hands on upper back of person.

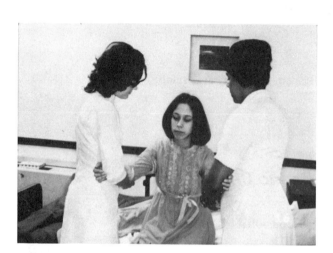

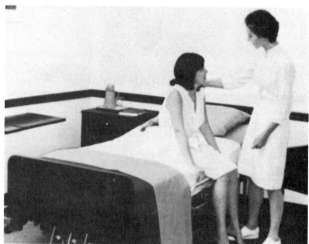

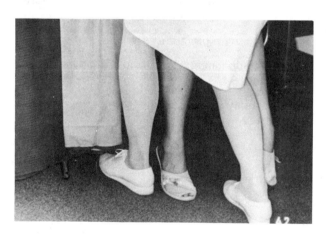

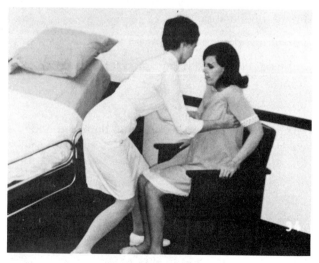

Pivot person toward chair on signal.

Gently lower person to chair.

Adjust position.

Align for safety with back to seat and leg touching chair. Avoid twisting your body and bending your back to prevent muscle strain.

Nurse flexes hips and knees to equalize effort over large muscles.

Use footrest or stool as needed.

Modifications and Other Considerations

For right hemiplegia, position chair at the foot of the bed. This places the unaffected left extremity toward the chair for safe pivot and easier sitting. If it is necessary to transfer from the other side of bed, place a chair at the head of the bed. A principle to follow is that with the person standing, the chair is placed so the seat will be at the person's unaffected side (Fig. III-1).

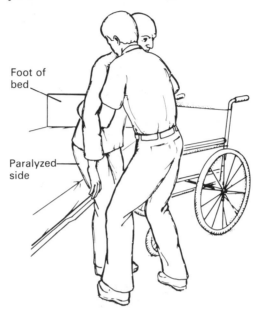

Foot of bed

Paralyzed side

Figure III-1
Assisting a person with hemiplegia from bed to chair

Note that for left hemiplegia, the above positioning is reversed. Figure III-2 shows a person with left hemiplegia transferring independently. Again, the wheelchair is positioned to enable the person to safely pivot on his unaffected leg.

For a casted lower extremity, place a chair parallel to the bed on the *affected* side, with chair and bed locked. You may stand against the chair at the far side and use your hands to support the cast while the person is using his hands secured on chair arms to pull and lift into chair (Fig. III-3).

Some persons at home or patients in institutions may use a mechanical lift, depending on extenuating circumstances.

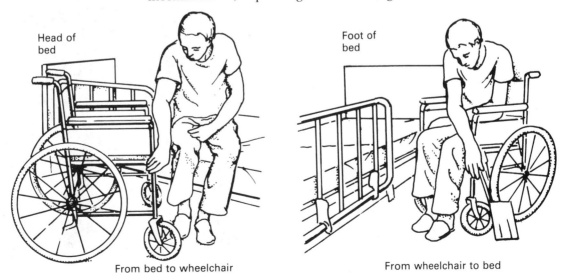

Head of bed

Foot of bed

From bed to wheelchair

From wheelchair to bed

Figure III-2
Persons with hemiplegia can transfer independently.

Figure III-3
Transferring from bed to chair with a cast

Procedure for Assisting a Person to Ambulate

Key Steps

Identify need for ambulation and modifications necessary.

Arrange suitable environment and supplies.

Assist person to sit and then dangle legs at bedside.

Discussion

Consult physician's orders and nursing-care plan. Assess general condition of person to tolerate procedure. Arrange suitable time for activity.

Obtain needed IV poles, robe, and slippers, and check environment for safety hazards.

Observe person's tolerance.

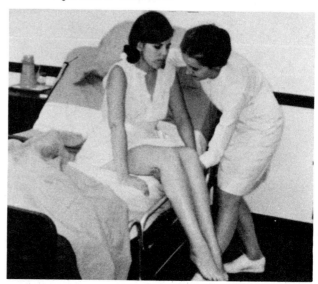

Key Steps

Assist person to standing position.

Assess person's stability and tolerance to stand erect at bedside.

Provide physical support for person while walking.

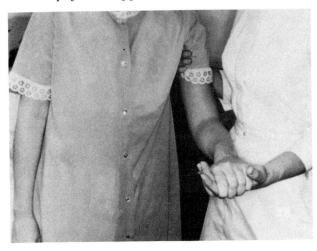

Return person to bed.

Modifications and Other Considerations

Discussion

Follow steps for assisting person from bed to chair.

Encouraging person to hold head up aids trunk balance. If faintness is more than momentary, return person to dangling position.

Nurse walks in rhythm at person's side with arm around waist or arm in arm. If person should become faint, ease yourself and person to floor to avoid injury.
Support for the person with an abdominal incision will facilitate standing straight. Build tolerance over time, walking only a few steps the first time.

Stand person at bed, dangle, and return to sitting then lying position.

A wide waistband called a walking belt is sometimes useful. The nurse provides security by holding handles at the back and sides as person ambulates.
Canes and walkers provide additional support for long-term assistance to the ambulating person.
If the person is extremely weakened or encumbered by equipment such as IVs, additional assistance will be needed.

Nutrition

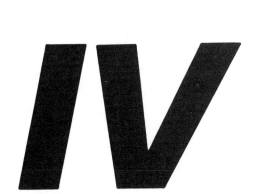

Nutrition, including the ability to ingest, absorb, and utilize food, is a basic need of all people. When normal nutrition is interrupted, the ability to meet higher-level needs is affected. Nurses need to be sensitive to unmet needs such as esteem or love and belonging when caring for individuals with altered nutrition. Some conditions that result in interruption in normal nutrition include surgery, problems of the head and neck (such as tumors), problems of the gastrointestinal tract (such as vomiting), or coma. This section describes procedures for persons needing mouth care, gastrointestinal decompression, and tube feedings.

Assessment of the Abdomen

Nurses need to be able to assess gastrointestinal function as one means of estimating nutritional status. For instance, abdominal assessment helps to determine the needs of an individual experiencing gastric decompression, or to recognize when diet changes may be indicated following surgery. In order to do an assessment of the abdomen, you must first identify the boundaries of the abdomen, including the xiphoid process, the costal margins, and the iliac crests (Fig. IV-1).

When assessing the abdomen, provide for privacy, and explain the procedure and its purpose. Expose the person's abdomen, and observe the skin for hydration, old scars, and rashes or discoloration. Next, observe the contour of the abdomen for symmetry, and note whether distention is present.

Auscultate the abdomen. Imagine a vertical line and a horizontal line passing through the umbilicus that divide the abdomen into four quadrants (see Fig. IV-1). Listen with your stethoscope for 1 full minute in each quadrant. You should hear 5 to 12 low-pitched, gurgling bowel sounds per minute.

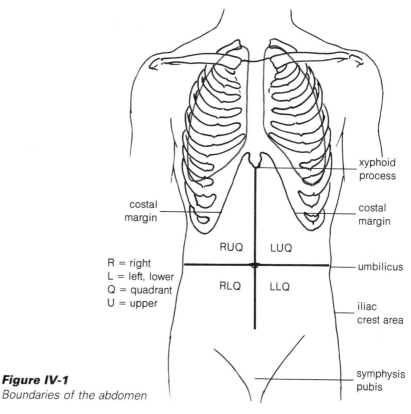

Figure IV-1
Boundaries of the abdomen

Percuss all four quadrants. The note produced is normally low pitched and hollow in most areas. In the right upper quadrant (RUQ) you will obtain a high-pitched, flat thud over the liver. A dull thud in other quadrants may indicate the presence of fluid, such as in a distended bladder, or a solid mass, such as a tumor. Finally, palpate lightly over the entire abdomen. It should be soft, except over bony areas. A firm, taut abdomen may indicate intestinal distention. Further discussion of abdominal assessment may be found in the text that accompanies this manual.

Mouth Care

Objectives

The student will provide mouth care to the client for the following purposes:

1 To moisturize and lubricate oral mucous membranes
2 To clean the teeth by removing food particles, bacteria, and other debris, using brushing and rinsing actions
3 To stimulate the gingivae
4 To provide a fresh feeling of the oral cavity

Introduction

A clean fresh mouth is essential for a sense of health and well-being. All persons, including those who are dependent, should be assisted to achieve adequate mouth care.

The most important action in the cleaning process is the mechanical action of brushing. Next in importance is the rinsing of the mouth with water.

Mouth washes and lemon–glycerine swabs may be used in between brushings but should not be used exclusive of brushing.

Procedure for Mouth Care

Key Steps

Wash hands.

Assemble the following equipment:

• Towel
• Kidney basin
• Toothbrush
• Dentifrice
• Cup of water or mouthwash
• Dental floss
• Petroleum jelly (Vaseline) or other lubricant

Position person.
Independent person:
Elevate head of bed 90°, and place overbed tray so person can reach supplies and be in a comfortable position to do own mouth care.

Discussion

Prevents spread of microorganisms.

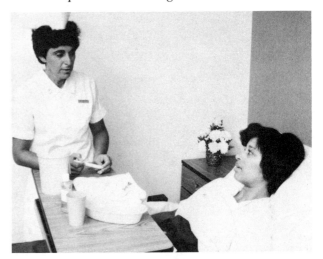

Key Steps   **Discussion**

Dependent or comatose person:
Elevate head of bed 30° and turn person on side
to prevent aspiration.

Brush teeth.
  Independent person:
  Assist as needed.

  Dependent or comatose person: Loosen food particles, mucus, and bacteria to
  Brush inner, outer, and chewing surfaces of all   decrease plaque build-up.
  teeth using moistened tooth brush and denti-   Mechanical action helps break up plaque and
  frice.   stimulate gums.
  Move brush over surfaces of teeth and gums in a   Take care to stimulate gums gently.
  small vibrating or circular motion.   Avoid areas with cracks or ulcerations.

  Brush bottom teeth upward from gum line and   Move debris from gum line toward external portion
  top teeth downward from gum line.   of the mouth.

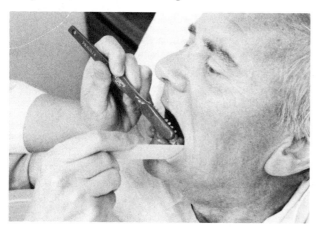

Rinse mouth vigorously with water three or four   Person can swish water around mouth and emit
times.   into kidney basin.

For the comatose or dependent person, rinse with
a bulb or plunger syringe and small amounts of
water. Suction water quickly to prevent aspiration.
Rinse three or four times.

Floss teeth.
  Independent person:
  Assist as needed.

  Dependent person:
  Insert floss between all teeth using a gentle saw-
  ing motion to break up and remove the debris
  caught between teeth.

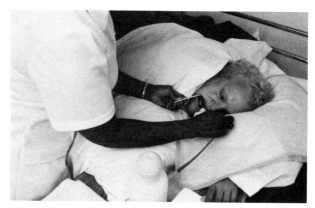

  Insert floss to just above gum line.   Prevents damage to the gingivae.

Apply petroleum jelly or other lubricant to the lips
to prevent cracking and flaking.

Do mouth care in the morning and evening, and   Assess individual person's needs.
more often as needed.

Key Steps   **Discussion**

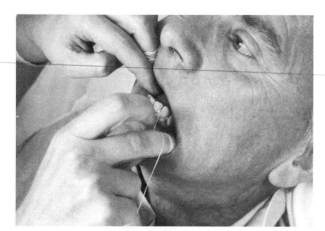
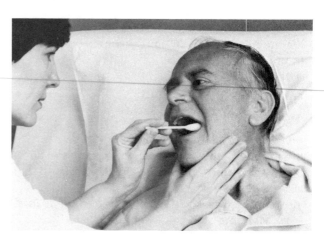

Modifications and Other Considerations

Use caution when assisting persons with lesions of the mouth to avoid further damage to oral mucous membranes. Normal saline or a half-and-half combination of water and hydrogen peroxide may be useful for mouth rinsing with these persons. However, the nurse will want to assess which solution is most comfortable.

Persons who have nasogastric tubes or are NPO for other reasons, those receiving oxygen therapy, and those who breathe primarily through the mouth will need more frequent mouth care.

Dentures, if worn, are best cleaned after they are removed from the mouth. Dentures may be soaked in lukewarm or cool water to loosen debris. Hold dentures firmly, and then brush in manner similar to that used for regular teeth. Have person rinse mouth with mouth wash, saline, or equal parts of water and hydrogen peroxide. Mouth may also be swabbed with lemon-glycerine swabs. Return teeth to person's mouth following cleaning procedure.

Decompression of the Gastrointestinal Tract

Objectives

The student will be able to do the following:

1 Identify four different tubes used for decompression.
2 Describe the procedure for inserting a nasogastric tube.
3 Identify five methods for determining placement of a nasogastric tube.
4 Identify the procedure for irrigating a nasogastric tube.
5 Provide care for persons experiencing gastric decompression.

Introduction

Decompression is the drainage of a person's stomach or small intestine by means of suction apparatus. Gastric or intestinal decompression is performed to prevent vomiting or distention of the gastrointestinal tract for persons at risk, such as in the postoperative period or in someone with bowel obstruction. Decompression is also used to obtain stomach contents for diagnostic purposes or to remove ingested, harmful substances such as in poisoning.

Tubes that are used for decompression are inserted through the nares and into the stomach or small intestine. There are four types of tubes for decompression: Levin, Salem, Cantor, and Miller–Abbott tubes.

Levin Tube

The Levin tube is used for decompression of the stomach or to provide a route for feeding. It is about 3 feet long. It has a number of holes at the tip and along the sides for the first 6 inches. This end of the tube (distal) is placed in the stomach, and the contents are drained through the holes. The proximal end of the tube extends about 10 inches out of the nares and may be connected to a suction machine or the tube-feeding equipment.

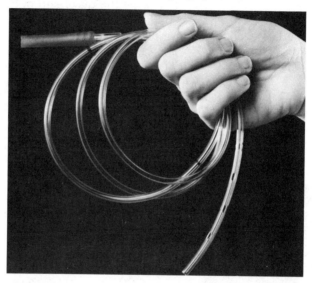

Salem Sump Tube

The Salem sump tube is used for decompression of the stomach and upper portion of the duodenum. This tube is similar to the Levin tube, except that it has another small "pigtail"-like tube extending out from its side. This second tube provides another lumen and is called a vent tube. The vent tube is a safety mechanism in that it prevents the development of excessive negative pressure and trauma to gastric mucosa should the gastric mucosa be sucked into the suction ports. The vent tube normally gives off a soft hissing sound, the absence of which may indicate that the lumen is clogged. In this case, irrigate the suction (large) tube. If gastric contents escape through the vent tube, both the suction lumen and the vent lumen should be irrigated. To prevent reflux of gastric drainage through the vent lumen, place vent lumen above patient's midline.

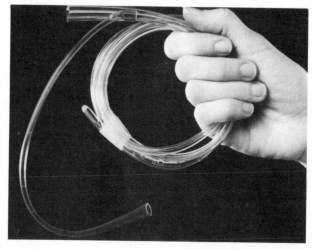

Cantor Tube

The Cantor tube is used for decompression of the small intestine. There is a small inflatable bag at the distal end of the tube, which is injected with 5 ml to 10 ml of mercury. The mercury provides weight, which helps the tube move along the intestine to the ileum and also assists in holding the tube in place in the ileum. The holes in this tube are at the proximal end of the bag. The proximal end of the tube is usually attached to a suction machine.

Miller–Abbott Tube

The Miller–Abbott tube is a double-lumen tube and is used for decompression of the small intestine. One lumen supplies the drainage passageway; the other lumen supplies an air passage to inflate the balloon at the distal end of the tube. The inflated balloon stimulates peristalsis and promotes passage of the tube through the intestine.

The same basic technique is used to insert all tubes. The insertion may be performed by a physician or a nurse, depending on institutional policy. Check the policy manual of your particular setting.

Decompression requires the use of suction following insertion of the tube. Usually a thermotic pump will be used. This electric pump provides intermittent suction through pressure changes produced by expanding and contracting air as it is alternately heated and cooled.

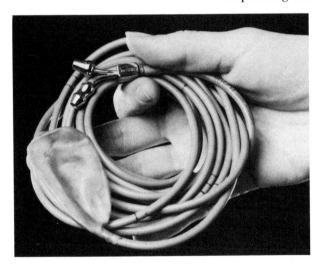

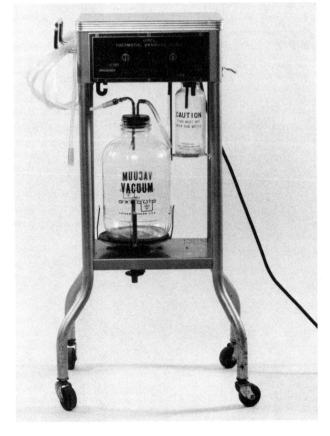

Procedure for Inserting a Nasogastric Tube

Key Steps	*Discussion*
Gather the following equipment:	

- Nasogastric (NG) tube
- Basin of ice
- Water soluble lubricant
- Glass of water and straw
- Stethoscope
- 30-ml syringe
- Tape

Explain procedure to person. Include in explanation what sensations might be experienced during the insertion and ways in which the person can ease the discomfort of insertion.	Elicits cooperation, and eases anxiety. Anxiety can cause muscle tension, which makes insertion of tube more difficult.
Approximate length of tubing for insertion. Place end of NG tube at tip of person's nose, to tip of ear lobe, and then to the end of the xiphoid process. Mark this length on the tube or note tube marking at this distance.	Provides length guide for proper placement of tube into stomach.

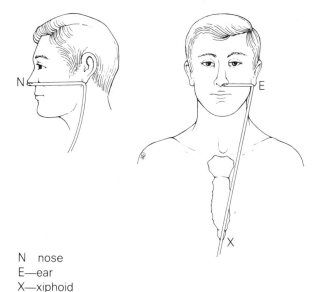

N   nose
E—ear
X—xiphoid

Chill tube in ice. Tube should be slightly stiffened and cold.	Assists in anesthetizing membrane linings. Prevents tube from curling in person's throat.
Lubricate end of tube with either water-soluble jelly or water.	Eases insertion, and prevents trauma to passageways. If tube is accidentally inserted into trachea, non-water-soluble lubricant might cause oil aspiration pneumonia.
Place person in high-Fowler's postion if person's condition permits.	Provides optimum open passageway and gravity assistance for insertion.

Key Steps	Discussion
Select nostril for insertion by gauging strongest air flow. (Gently place your finger under both nostrils to feel air flow.)	Obstructed or narrowed nostrils increase difficulty and discomfort of insertion.
Insert tube gently but steadily. The person will gag when the tube reaches the posterior pharynx. Encourage the person to swallow (or sip water if condition permits), and continue gentle steady insertion. Encourage mouth breathing and continued swallowing.	Gagging reflex is temporary and will subside when tube has passed posterior pharynx. Persistent gagging may indicate too fast or too slow insertion. Directs tube into esophagus as swallowing closes the epiglottis, preventing insertion into the trachea.
Confirm placement of tube in the stomach when measurement mark is reached. Use one or more of the following methods:	Prevents complications from improper tube placement.
• Observe the person for signs of respiratory distress, cyanosis, or chest pain.	These signs may indicate that the tube has entered the trachea or lungs.
• Aspirate the tube with syringe. If the tube is in the stomach, you may be able to aspirate stomach contents.	Return gastric contents to the stomach following aspiration to prevent possible electrolyte imbalance.
• Place a stethoscope over the epigastric area while injecting 10 ml to 30 ml of air with a syringe. A "whoosh" should be heard as the air enters the stomach.	The "whoosh" is difficult to hear on some people; therefore, this method should be used along with at least one of the other methods for confirming placement.
• Hold proximal end of tube up to your face to feel for an air flow.	An air flow could indicate the tube has entered the respiratory tract.
• Ask the person to inhale and hold breath. Place proximal end of tube in a glass of water. Then ask the person to exhale. If the tube has entered the respiratory tract, there will be bubbling in the water.	This method should be used with caution. If the tube is in the respiratory tract, it will function as a straw if the person inhales while the proximal end is placed in water. Positioning the cup of water below the level of the person's chest while performing this method decreases the risk of aspiration.
Secure tape around tube and in criss-cross fashion on bridge of nose.	Proper taping prevents discomfort of friction and complication of nasal skin breakdown. Helps maintain proper tube placement.
Position person in semi-Fowler's position if person's condition permits.	Prevents reflux of gastric secretions into esophagus, which yields sensation of "heartburn."

Procedure for Gastric Decompression

Key Steps	Discussion
Provide person with explanation and information of what to expect while NG tube is in place and decompression is occurring.	Be aware of the altered body image that the person with an NG tube may experience. Consider that the person may have just had an uncomfortable experience with tube insertion, may have had an uncomfortable past experience with an NG tube, or

Key Steps

Discussion

may be apprehensive because of lack of familiarity with the tube.

Prepare suction pump for operation as follows:

- Plug pump into an outlet.
- Set pressure correctly and according to physician's order.

Usually only low-pressure, intermittent suction is used because excessive negative pressure, either in the stomach or the bowel, may pull the mucosa into the sucking ports of the tube. With Salem sump tubes, constant rather than intermittent suction should be used. Intermittent suction with these double-lumen NG tubes decreases the efficiency of the tube and allows gastric drainage to escape by the vent tube. Institutional policies vary and should be checked.

- Check connections of tubes and bottle cap in collection bottle to be sure they are intact and airtight.

Any air leak will cause an interruption in pressure and inefficient suctioning.

Check suction pump before connecting to NG tube. Turn switch to "on," and place drainage tube in a cup of premeasured water; if the water is sucked up, the machine is functioning.

Be sure to subtract the amount of water used from the contents in the collection bottle to ensure an accurate measurement of output.

Connect drainage tube of suction pump to NG tube.

Be sure this junction is also airtight.

Check the amount of drainage, and record at least every 8 hours.

Observe the amount, color, consistency, and odor of the drainage. The frequency of observation is dependent on the person's needs.
Normal gastric contents are a yellow green mucoid material. The normal gastric contents from an empty stomach are a clear, mucoid liquid.

When signs that indicate either a malfunctioning suction machine or clogged tube are present, proceed with the following:

A few of these signs are: person vomits around NG tube; person complains of nausea; no NG drainage; abdominal distention.

- Check tube for placement.
- Check suction pump.
- Irrigate tube with 30 ml of normal saline as ordered.
- Lastly, reposition person or tube to facilitate drainage.

Also check drainage tube for clogs by disconnecting at junction of NG tube and "milking" the tube toward bottle. This may assist in dislodging any obstruction in the tube itself. If, after checking tube placement, suction pump and irrigation, it still fails to drain, the sucking ports of the tube may be occluded by gastric mucosa.
Do not manipulate the tube if it was placed during a surgical procedure, so as not to intrude on the suture line. Notify the physician.

Provide skin care around nares where tube is inserted by doing the following:

This will prevent nasal skin breakdown. If the skin becomes irritated, lubricate with water-soluble lubricant or rosewater ointment.

- Keep area clean and dry
- Change tape as necessary.

When retaping, move tube slightly on nares and secure in a different position.

Key Steps	Discussion
Provide mouth care a minimum of three times per day as follows: • Brush teeth. • Apply water-soluble lubricant or rosewater ointment to lips. • Give cracked ice or throat lozenges.	This will assist in preventing dryness of the oral cavity and pharynx. It is necessary to obtain a physician's order for these measures.
Be alert to complaints of upper left quadrant abdominal pain. This could indicate irritation to the gastric mucosa. • Instruct the person to turn frequently from side to side. • Advance or retract the tube 2 inches or 3 inches. • The physician may order an antacid to be inserted through the tube.	 Remember, if the person has had a surgery where the tube was placed during the surgical procedure to prevent intrusion on the suture line, do not manipulate the tube. Following the administration of the antacid, the tube is clamped for 30 minutes.

Procedure for Irrigating a Nasogastric Tube

A nasogastric (NG) tube is irrigated for the following reasons:
- To check for patency
- To flush the tubing for cleanliness
- To dislodge any material that may be clogging the tube and its sucking ports

A physician's order is necessary to irrigate the NG tube. The order will usually designate the amount and solution to be used. In general, an NG tube may be irrigated with 30 ml of normal saline, tap water, or air. You may find that institutions differ in their procedures concerning the use of air for irrigation.

Key Steps	Discussion
Gather the following equipment: • Graduated container • Irrigation solution • Syringe	
Explain procedure to the person.	This will assist in decreasing any fears. There is generally no sensation experienced with this procedure.
Pour irrigation solution into graduated container.	Amount of solution may be specified by physician.
Disconnect NG tube from the drainage tubing.	Maintain cleanliness of drainage tube by securing to side of the suction pump.
Remove bulb or plunger from syringe, and insert tip of syringe into NG tube.	To ensure accurate intake and output records, record the amounts of irrigating solution instilled. Unless an equal amount of the solution is aspirated by syringe, subtract the amount not aspirated from the total amount of gastric drainage.

Key Steps

Pour solution into syringe, and allow the fluid to flow in by gravity.

Reinsert bulb or plunger, and aspirate irrigation solution back with syringe.

Record any discrepancies of fluid return and characteristics of the gastric contents.

Discussion

If NG tube is clogged, it may be necessary to reinsert bulb or plunger and apply gentle pressure.

Occasionally, negative pressure prevents the aspiration of the irrigation solution. Resistance or a pull is experienced when pulling back plunger of syringe. Do not force the aspiration. This may indicate that mucosa is obstructing the sucking ports of the tube. Repositioning the person or the tube may facilitate drainage. If NG tube was placed during the surgical procedure so as not to intrude on surgical line, notify the physician before manipulating the tube.

The characteristics to note are its color, character, and odor.

Modifications

The double-lumen Salem sump tube may require irrigation of both lumens. The vent tube will normally give off a hissing sound. When this is not present and gastric drainage begins escaping from the vent tube, the sucking lumen may be clogged and should be irrigated. Following irrigation, if gastric drainage is still leaking from the vent tube, irrigate and clear the vent tube itself. Although institutional policies may vary, usually 10 ml of saline followed by 10 ml to 20 ml of air is ordered.

Tube Feeding

Objectives

The student will be able to do the following:

1 Describe the purposes for administering a tube feeding.
2 Provide care for persons receiving nutrition by way of tube feeding.

Introduction

Tube feeding involves the administration of a liquid formula through a tube into the gastrointestinal tract. Tube feedings provide nutrition to persons who are unable to ingest food in the usual manner, including comatose or dysphagic individuals, those with painful lesions of the oral cavity, or people with fractured jaws. Tube feedings are also sometimes used to treat persons with anorexia nervosa.

   Any nutritious liquid can be administered during a tube feeding. Feedings may be blenderized and prepared within the home or institution, or they may be commercially prepared. Tube feedings can supply a nutritionally adequate and well-balanced diet.

   Tube feedings can be administered by two routes, nasogastric tube and gastrostomy tube (Fig. IV-2). The most common route involves a nasogastric tube, using a Levin tube (described in the previous section), which is passed through the nose, pharynx, esophagus, and into the stomach. Gastrostomy feeding involves placing a tube through a surgical incision in the abdominal wall into the stomach. The procedure for nasogastric and gastrostomy tube feedings is basically the same.

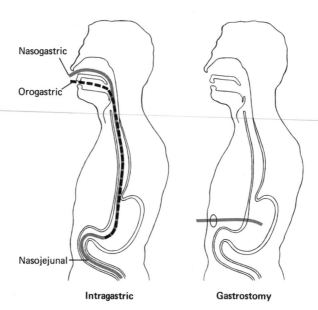

Nasogastric

Orogastric

Nasojejunal

Intragastric   **Gastrostomy**

Figure IV-2
Types and sites of gastric feeding.
Intragastric (nasogastric, NG): A tube is passed through the nose or mouth into the stomach and secured in place. (A tube passed through the mouth is more correctly called an orogastric tube. An orogastric tube is ordinarily inserted at mealtime and removed following the meal.) Intragastric tube preferred for short-term gavage feeding; easily inserted by physician or nurse, remains in place between feedings. (Some clients are taught to insert their own tube; they may remove the tube between meals.) Variations include nasopharyngeal and nasojejunal feeding tubes.
Gastrostomy: A temporary or permanent stoma is constructed allowing food to be introduced through the skin directly into the stomach. Preferred for long-term gavage feeding of children and for long-term feeding of adults when use of esophagus is contraindicated. Disadvantages: partial undressing necessary at mealtime; skin care may pose problems.

It is essential to determine the placement of nasogastric tubes prior to each feeding. Administration of feeding through a tube that is misplaced in the respiratory tract can be lethal.

Procedure for Administering a Tube Feeding

Key Steps	**Discussion**
Explain procedure to person.	This will ease anxiety and elicit cooperation.
Assemble necessary equipment as follows:	
• Syringe or gavage bag	A gavage bag is generally used when instilling larger amounts of formula.
• Formula	Liquified food, hospital-prepared blenderized tube feedings, or commercially prepared liquid formulas are a few of the preparations a physician may order.
• Graduated pitcher	
• IV pole (if using gavage bag)	

Key Steps

Measure formula into graduated pitcher. Warm to room temperature.

If using gavage bag, close clamp on gavage bag, and pour formula into bag. Open clamp and allow formula to flow until all air has been expelled from tubing.

Place person in high-Fowler's position.

Confirm placement of tube.

Aspirate gastric secretions. If able to aspirate more than 50 ml, withhold feeding and notify physician.

Connect tube to gavage bag or syringe, and begin the feeding.

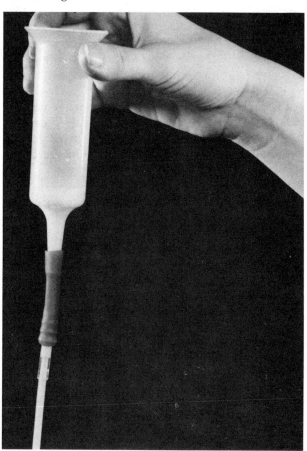

Discussion

Warming can be done either by removing formula from refrigeration ½ hour before feeding or by placing it in a container of warm water immediately before feeding. A person is better able to tolerate the feeding if it is at room temperature.

Prevents air from entering stomach, which causes distention.

Facilitates by gravity the administration of feeding into the stomach.

Prevents administration of formula into respiratory tract. Methods for confirming tube placement are discussed under Insertion of Nasogastric Tubes, p 77. It is not necessary to confirm the placement of a gastrostomy tube because it is secured in the stomach.

Prevents gastric distention should the previous feeding not have been absorbed. Check institutional policies regarding replacing aspirate. Usually the aspirate is replaced to prevent electrolyte depletion.

With gavage bag, hang bag from IV pole and regulate the flow, according to the person's tolerance, by the clamp or by raising or lowering the bag. Normally, the flow will be a fast, steady drip over 20 minutes to ½ hour. When using a syringe, remove the plunger or bulb, insert the tip of the

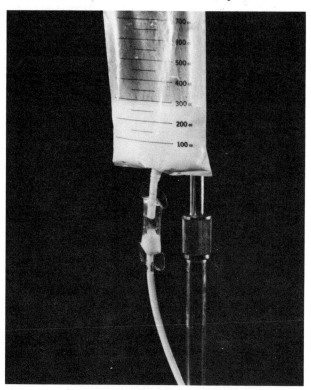

Key Steps

Discussion

syringe into the tube, and pour the formula into the syringe so that the feeding flows in by gravity. The syringe is held by hand, and flow rate can be regulated by raising or lowering the syringe. The syringe is refilled until feeding is completed.

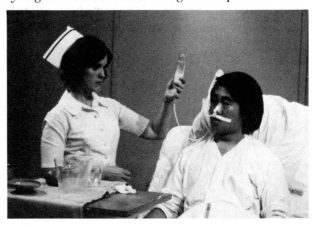

Observe the person throughout the feeding for signs of intolerance. Signs of intolerance will be complaints of cramping or nausea, or abdominal distention. Stop the procedure immediately if the person shows signs of discomfort.

Following the feeding, flush the tube with 30 ml to 50 ml of tap water.

This provides patency and cleanliness and prevents bacterial growth in the tube.

Clamp the tube, and continue the high-Fowler's position for 30 minutes.

If high-Fowler's position is not possible, position the person on his right side with head elevated. These positions encourage the stomach to empty and discourage regurgitation.

Record the time, amount, and type of formula given and the person's tolerance to the procedure.

Provides documentation.

Other Considerations

The person receiving tube feedings often experiences altered body image related to the presence of the feeding tube and the unnatural eating method. The person should be helped to explore his feelings about the presence of the tube, and the nurse should provide companionship during feeding times. Tube feedings may result in dry mouth, nasal skin breakdown, or irritation to the gastric mucosa. See Procedure for Gastric Decomposition, p 78, for interventions for these problems.

Oral medications may be administered by way of nasogastric or gastrostomy tubes. Dilute a medication with about 30 ml of water so that it will flow easily through the tube, and administer it with a syringe. Flush the tube with 30 ml of water or more after administering the medication to clear the tubing. If fluids must be restricted, an alternative method is to flush the tubing with 30 ml of air. Be sure to check the placement of the nasogastric tube each time prior to administering a medication.

Elimination

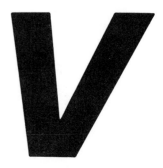

Elimination refers to the function of the bowel and urinary system. Persons at risk for problems of elimination include individuals undergoing surgery, those on bed rest, persons with neurological dysfunction, and those with diseases of the bowel or urinary tract. This section presents specific skills for assessing elimination function and maintaining or restoring normal elimination, such as catheterization, catheter irrigation, enema administration, stoma care, and colostomy irrigation. Because control of elimination is learned early in life and the act is considered private, loss of function often causes alterations in body image and feelings of shame. Thus, nurses assist by being attentive to both the psychological and physiological implications of bowel and bladder problems.

Urinary Catheterization

Objectives

The student will be able to do the following:

1 Identify several reasons for urinary catheterization.

2 Describe the hazards of urinary catheterization.

3 Place catheter into the bladder using sterile technique.

Introduction

Urinary catheterization is the introduction of a catheter through the urethra and into the bladder in order to remove urine. Some of the reasons for catheterization of the bladder include the following:

- To prevent accidental incision into a distended bladder during and after surgery of the abdominal area

- To relieve bladder distention in persons experiencing urinary retention or urethral obstruction

- To allow frequent monitoring of urine (such as in diabetic keto-acidosis, shock, or following kidney transplants)

- To prevent radiation burns of the bladder in women treated with radium implant in the vagina

- To provide temporary control of bladder elimination for persons who have lost neuromuscular control of voiding reflex

A potential for infection is always present during and after catheterization and is the greatest risk involved in this procedure. The bladder is normally a sterile cavity. However, microorganisms may be introduced into the bladder with a contaminated catheter. The catheter also provides a direct pathway for bacteria to travel into the bladder. It is important that strict aseptic technique be used during and after the procedure.

Trauma to the bladder and urethra can also occur as a result of catheterization. Friction, as the catheter is passed, can irritate the mucous membrane lining the urethra. The bladder and urethra can be punctured if the catheter is forced through a stricture or curve as it is being passed.

Another hazard may result from rapid decompression of an overdistended bladder, leading to systemic reactions such as chills or shock. No more than 750 ml to 1000 ml of urine should be withdrawn from the bladder at a time.

Types of Catheters

You will see two types of catheters used frequently (Fig. V-1). The first type is the straight catheter (also called a French or Robinson catheter) that consists of a single-lumen tube. This type of catheter is used when the person is catheterized for a urine specimen or relief of urinary retention. The catheter will not be left in place for continuous drainage.

The second type is the Foley catheter (also called an indwelling or retention catheter). It is used when continuous drainage of urine is necessary. The Foley catheter has a double lumen. One lumen allows urine to flow from the bladder into the collecting device. The second lumen opens at a side piece and ends at a balloon near the tip of the catheter. After the catheter is in the bladder, water, air, or saline is introduced into the side piece with a syringe. This distends the balloon making it larger than the urethral opening and prevents the catheter from slipping out of the bladder. The side piece is self-sealing so the fluid or air will not leak out of the balloon once it is inflated. The various balloons will hold from 5 ml to 30 ml of fluid or air. The amount the balloon holds is marked on the side piece.

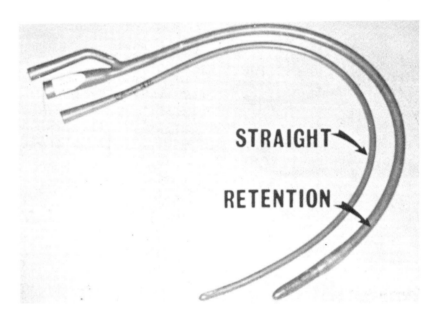

Figure V-I
Straight and retention catheters

Catheters come in different sizes indicated by numbers (French calibrations). The larger the number, the larger is the lumen. The most commonly used sizes are the following:

#8–#10	Children
#14–#16	Women
#16–#20	Men

The size of the catheter is also marked on the side piece of the Foley-type catheter.

Collection Devices

Persons who have continuous drainage of the bladder require a device for collection of urine from the catheter. The dependent drainage bag serves this purpose. The bag, which is plastic and disposable, connects to the catheter by means of plastic tubing. Another piece of tubing at the bottom of the bag allows it to be emptied without disconnecting it from the catheter. Graduated markings indicate the amount of urine in the bag. These markings are only approximate, however. Urine should always be emptied from the bag and measured with a graduated container to determine the volume accurately.

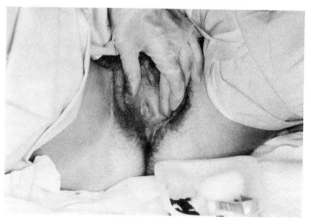

Leg bags are also available for persons who need long-term catheterization. They attach to the leg by straps and are unobtrusive under clothing.

Anatomical Considerations

The main problem in catheterizing a woman is locating the urinary meatus. It can be found between the labia minora, above the vagina, and below the clitoris. It can be distinguished from the vaginal opening by its small size. The urinary meatus is best located by separating the labia and gently pulling upward toward the symphysis pubis (Fig. V-2).

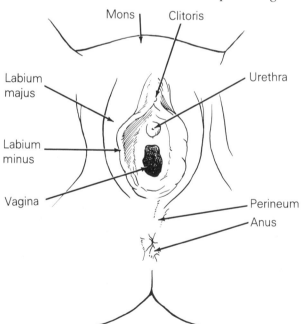

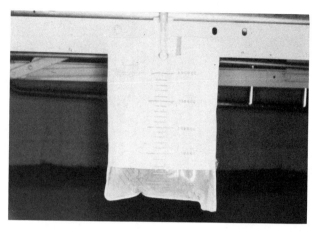

Figure V-2
Diagram and photo of female external genitalia

In men, the length and curvature of the urethra present the main difficulty in catheterization. The urethra is approximately 8 inches long and makes several curves before ending in the urinary bladder (Fig. V-3). By holding the penis vertical to the long axis of the body during insertion of the catheter, these curvatures are straightened. Resistance at the fossa navicularis and vesical sphincter can be overcome by asking the man to breathe through his mouth (to promote relaxation) and by twisting the catheter slightly as it is being inserted.

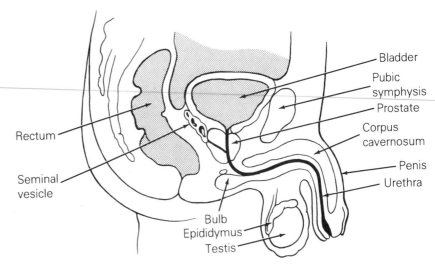

Figure V-3
Male genitourinary tract

Procedure for Urinary Catheterization of the Female (Indwelling Catheter)

Key Steps

Gather the following equipment:
- Catheterization tray
- Catheter (if needed)
- Bath blanket
- Light source

Explain the procedure to the person. Tell her why the procedure is being done and what it will achieve.

Wash hands.

Provide privacy.

Position person in the dorsal recumbent position with legs spread apart and knees flexed. This position allows easiest means for identifying the urinary meatus.

Discussion

Most institutions use sterile, prepackaged catheterization sets that contain all of the necessary equipment. Some do not contain catheters or may contain the wrong size.

Decreases anxiety. Anxiety may cause muscle tension, which will make insertion of the catheter difficult.

Decreases the spread of microorganisms.

Protects the person from embarrassment.

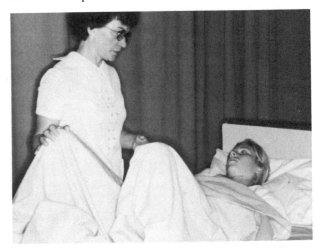

Secure lighting so that perineal area is illuminated.

Cover person's legs with bath blanket.

Protects the person from unnecessary exposure. Protects the bedding from soiling.

Key Steps

Open catheterization kit.

Position underpad under person's buttocks, plastic side down. Handle pad only by corners.

Position drape (with hole) over the perineal area, keeping the labia exposed through the hole.

If kit does not contain a catheter, open separate catheter package and drop catheter on sterile field.

Put on sterile gloves to prevent introduction of microorganisms from hands into the bladder.

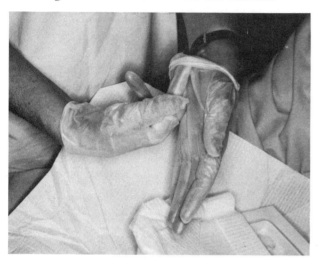

Open the package of antiseptic solution and pour over cotton balls.

Open package of lubricating jelly and apply to first 3 inches of the catheter to decrease friction between the catheter and urethra.

Remove cap from the tip of the syringe and connect to side piece of catheter.

Place tray containing equipment on sterile pad between person's legs.

Connect catheter to dependent drainage bag.

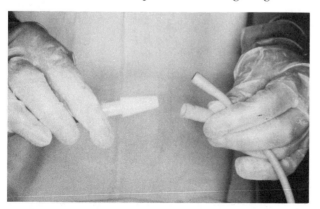

Discussion

Provides a sterile field.

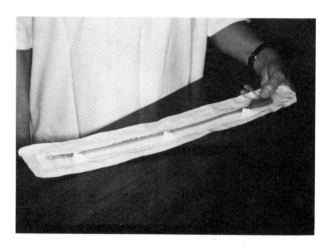

Do prior to catheterization so that if you enter full bladder you do not lose urine.

Key Steps

Discussion

With left hand, separate labia and pull upward. (Use right hand if you are left handed.) Identify the meatus; keep this hand in place during the rest of the procedure. It is no longer sterile.

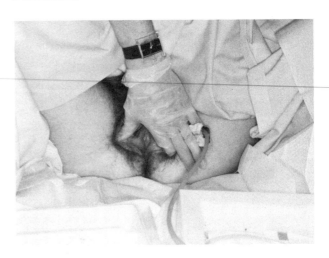

With plastic forceps, pick up a cotton ball and cleanse the area around the meatus. Using one stroke, wipe from meatus toward the anus and dispose of the cotton ball (not on your sterile field). Repeat with remaining cotton balls.

Decreases introduction of microorganisms into bladder. Prevents wiping microorganisms from anus into area surrounding the meatus.

Pick up catheter near the tip with sterile hand. Slowly insert catheter through meatus 2 inches to 4 inches (female urethra is 1½ inches to 2 inches long) until urine appears through the catheter.

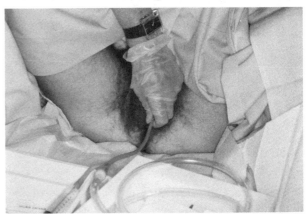

Once urine appears in catheter, insert it an additional ½ inch. Have the person breathe through the mouth or "pant" while catheter is being inserted. Indicate that she will feel slight pressure as catheter passes the sphincter.

Ascertains that catheter has passed through urethra and into bladder.
Minimizes anxiety and relaxes sphincter and perineal muscles.

Continue to grasp catheter with one hand. Slowly inject the required amount of water or air to inflate the balloon. If the person complains of pain while you are doing this, deflate the balloon and insert the catheter further into the bladder. Now start inflating the balloon again.

Balloon may be in the patient's urethra. Further inflation may result in trauma.

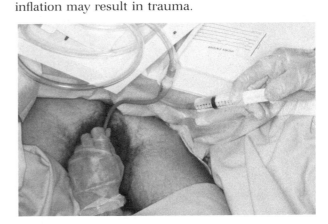

Key Steps

Remove syringe from side piece. Apply slight pull on the catheter. You should feel resistance to your pull.

Remove gloves. Tape catheter to the person's thigh. This prevents irritation and infection from catheter sliding in urethra. Also prevents trauma from accidental pulling on drainage tubing.

Chart the time of catheterization and amount and characteristics of urine obtained.

Discussion

Ascertains that the catheter is secure in the bladder.

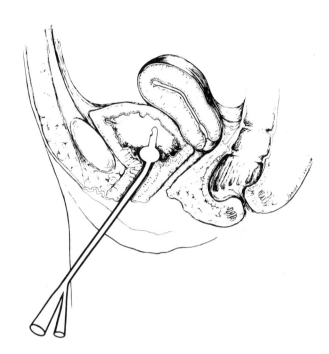

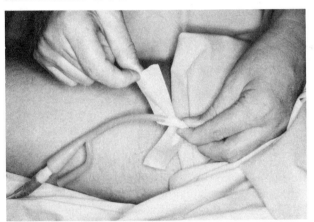

Modifications

Male Catheterization

The procedure for catheterization of a man is identical to that of a woman. You will need to hold the penis at a right angle to the long axis of the body with one hand. This will straighten the natural curvature of the urethra. You will need to insert the catheter approximately 8 inches to 9 inches through the urethra before inflating the balloon.

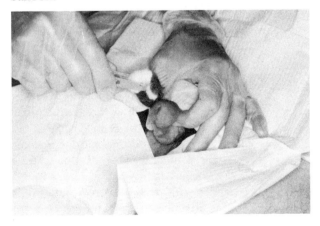

Straight Catheter

To insert a straight (non-indwelling) catheter follow the procedure outlined above, but omit the steps that refer to inflating the balloon.

Self-Catheterization

Some individuals, particularly those with neurological deficits, partial urethral obstruction, or temporary inability to micturate, may be taught to catheterize themselves. Intermittent self-catheterization (ISC) is performed using clean, rather than sterile, technique. The rationale for use of clean technique is that urinary tract infections in persons with overdistended bladders result from tissue injury and impaired bladder defense mechanisms rather than from introduction of bacteria into the bladder *per se.* The person will need to learn the procedure for straight catheterization as well as other measures directed toward prevention of urinary tract infection.

Irrigation of an Indwelling Catheter

Objectives

The student will be able to do the following:

1 Describe the purpose of bladder irrigation.

2 Irrigate an indwelling catheter using the closed and open methods.

Introduction

The purpose of bladder irrigation for anyone with an indwelling catheter is to cleanse the bladder or to maintain patency of the catheter.

This procedure is not done as frequently as in the past because of the danger of introducing microorganisms into the bladder. The best method of bladder irrigation is adequate fluid intake. Unless there is a fluid restriction, assist persons with an indwelling catheter to maintain an optimal fluid intake.

When a bladder irrigation is done, strict aseptic technique must be used. The solution to be used in the irrigation is ordered by the physician. Solutions that are used include normal saline, ¼% acetic acid, and commercial preparations. You will need to consult a drug reference book to check the composition of commercially prepared solutions.

There are two mechanical methods of catheter irrigation: the open method and the closed method. The procedures for each of these will be described below.

The open method of catheter irrigation involves disconnection of the catheter from the drainage tubing. This method should only be used when essential, because the potential for contamination of the urinary system is increased whenever the drainage system is opened. A bulb syringe is used for lavage. The type of lavage may be either "gentle" or "forceful" and is ordered by the physician.

The forceful method was used for many years and may still be necessary when there are clots of blood or mucus shreds present in the urine. The bulb syringe is used to gently force the irrigating solution into the bladder. Forceful lavage should only be used when essential, because trauma to the mucous lining of the bladder may occur.

In *the gentle method* the bulb syringe, without the rubber bulb, is attached to the catheter. The irrigation solution is poured directly into the syringe and will flow into the catheter by gravity. This is the preferable open-method procedure because it minimizes the chance of trauma associated with forceful lavage.

The closed method, currently the one of choice, minimizes the introduction of microorganisms into the urinary system. Because it is a more gentle procedure, it minimizes trauma to the mucous lining of the bladder as well.

Procedure for Closed Method of Catheter Irrigation

Key Steps

Gather the following equipment:

- Sterile 30-ml syringe
- 21 gauge, 1¼-inch needle
- Sterile 50 ml to 100 ml container
- 30 ml sterile normal saline
- Alcohol swabs

Wash hands.

Explain the procedure to the person.

Draw up 30 ml of irrigating solution into the syringe. Cap the needle until you are ready to irrigate.

Locate the connection of the catheter to the dependent drainage tubing. Note the 1-inch section between the point of connection and the bifurcation of the catheter. This is the point for needle insertion.

Discussion

Decreases potential for contamination.

Minimizes anxiety.

Prevents contamination of needle.

If a needle is inserted beyond the bifurcation, the lumen that inflates the balloon at the end of the catheter may be punctured. If the fluid leaks from the balloon and deflates it, the catheter will fall out.

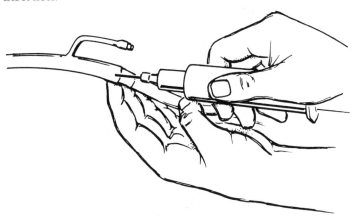

Do not disconnect catheter from drainage tubing.

Place a clamp on the plastic drainage tubing.

Prepare the needle insertion point with an alcohol swab.

Insert the needle at a 45° angle, taking care to penetrate one side of the catheter only, as shown above.

Maintenance of a closed system minimizes the entrance of bacteria into the urinary tract.

This ensures entrance of the irrigating solution into the bladder and prevents it from entering the drainage bag.

Reduces the number of bacteria on the catheter area.

Insertion of the needle at a 45° angle will cause minimal damage to the latex catheter. This material is designed to reseal itself after being punctured.

Key Steps

Slowly instill the fluid. Indicate to the person that it may feel cold as it enters.

Wthdraw the needle.

Release the clamp on the drainage tubing.

Record amount of irrigation fluid instilled on the intake and output sheet in the output column. Label it as fluid instilled.

Chart the amount of fluid instilled, appearance of returned fluid, and person's response.

Discussion

Slow instillation produces minimal trauma to the mucous lining of the bladder. Informing the client of sensations minimizes anxiety.

The irrigation fluid will now drain freely (by gravity) into the drainage bag.

When the output for each shift is totaled, the amount of irrigation fluid instilled during that period should be subtracted from the output.

Open Method of Catheter Irrigation

Review the principles of sterile technique. Remember that any equipment that comes in direct contact with the irrigating solution, catheter, or collection bag tubing must be kept sterile. This includes the plastic portion of the bulb syringe, the inside of the squeeze bulb, the inside of the graduated container, and the 4 × 4 gauze pads used to cover the tubing from the collection bag.

Procedure for Open Catheter Irrigation—Forceful

Key Steps

Gather the following equipment:
- Sterile irrigation set containing bulb syringe
- Graduated container and collection basin
- Irrigating solution
- Sterile 4 × 4's
- Clamp
- Blue pad

Wash hands.

Explain to the person what you are going to do and the purpose of the irrigation.

Provide for privacy, and position person comfortably.

Discussion

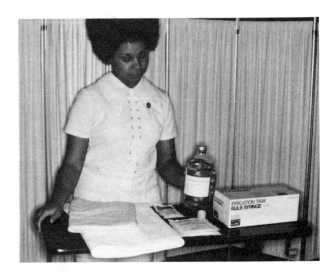

Decreases spread of microorganisms.

Decreases anxiety.

Protects the person from embarrassment.

Key Steps	**Discussion**
Expose the catheter. Position the blue pad on the bed under the working area.	Protects the bedding.
Remove cap from irrigating solution.	Prepares bottle for easy pouring when hand is gloved.
Open irrigation tray, keeping inside of wrapper sterile.	Provides sterile working field.
Remove syringe from container handling by the bulb and hold in one hand.	Be careful not to touch other parts of the syringe to maintain sterility of equipment.
With empty hand, pour required amount of solution into irrigating bottle. Measure accurately the amount of solution you pour into container.	Maintain accurate output record.
Return syringe to container.	

Hold catheter tubing upright to allow urine to flow into bag and to maintain sterility of catheter and tubing ends. Disconnect tubing from catheter without touching either end to prevent introduction of microorganisms into the bladder.

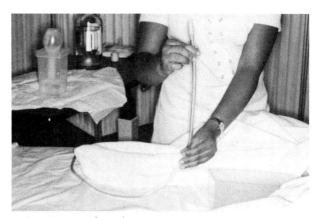

Hook catheter into slot on irrigation tray.

Maintains sterility.

Cover end of tubing with sterile 4 × 4, and clamp. Immobilize this tubing by taping it to bed or stand.

Maintains sterility.
Clamp prevents leakage of urine.

Fill the syringe with irrigation solution as follows:

- Hold the syringe out of the bottle, and squeeze the bulb to eject air and to prevent the solution from splashing or overflowing.
- Continue to squeeze the bulb, and insert syringe into irrigation fluid.
- Release grasp on bulb.
- Syringe will fill with solution.

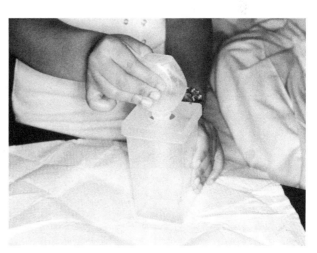

Place tip of syringe firmly into the end of catheter. Gently squeeze the bulb to inject fluid into the bladder. Gentle pressure prevents trauma to the mucous lining of the bladder.

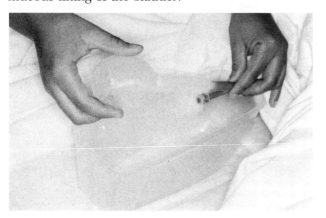

Key Steps   **Discussion**

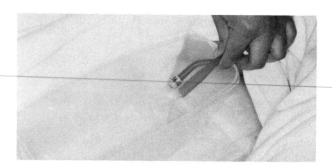

Maintain squeeze on bulb and remove syringe. Allow solution to drain into irrigation tray by holding catheter downward. (Fluid flows in direction of gravity.) Repeat steps as necessary, until all solution is used or return is clear and free of shreds.

Remove 4 × 4 from collecting bag tubing and connect to the catheter without touching ends.

Reestablishes a closed drainage system. Maintains sterility of catheter and tubing ends and prevents entrance of microorganisms.

Measure the amount of fluid returned from the bladder by pouring the drainage from irrigation tray into solution container. If there is more fluid than you started with, subtract this amount from the output record.

Urine may have been drawn from the person's bladder during the irrigation.

Procedure for Open Catheter Irrigation—Gentle

Key Steps   **Discussion**

Follow procedure for forceful open method up to and including covering tubing and immobilizing it.

Maintains sterility of equipment and field.

Pick up syringe, grasping it high at neck, and remove bulb. Be careful not to touch tip of syringe. Place bulb, sterile end down, onto sterile field.

Place tip of syringe firmly into the end of the catheter. Slowly pour all the irrigating solution into the syringe and allow it to flow into the bladder by gravity.

Fluid flowing into the bladder by gravity produces the least amount of trauma to the mucous lining.

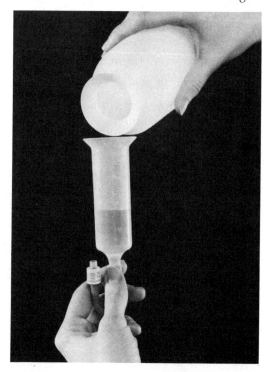

Key Steps	Discussion
If resistance is met, pick up bulb, connect to syringe, and gently squeeze.	Resistance may indicate catheter is clogged, and this will gently clear it.
Continue with last two steps of forceful open method.	

Urine Testing

Objectives

The student will be able to do the following:

1 Describe the procedure for obtaining a clean, midstream urine specimen.
2 Test urine for glucose, acetone, and specific gravity.

Introduction

Nurses often collect urine specimens and perform urine testing to assess the status of urinary elimination. Such collections often involve instructing the person how to obtain a clean urine specimen. Three of the most common urine tests are those for glucose, acetone, and specific gravity. Descriptions of each of these procedures are included in this section.

Clean-Catch Urine Specimen

Clean-catch specimens may also be called midstream urine specimens. Voided urine specimens may be contaminated by organisms present around the meatus. A bacteriologic examination performed on voided urine cannot distinguish between organisms present in the urinary tract and those which entered the urine from the external meatal area. It is possible, however, by means of the clean-catch specimen to achieve a reliable bacteriologic evaluation. This procedure also avoids the use, and thus the hazards, of catheterization.

Procedure for Obtaining a Clean-Catch Urine Specimen

Key Steps	Discussion
Female: Instruct the woman to do the following: • Separate labia to expose urethral orifice.	
• Cleanse around orifice with a sponge soaked in soap and water.	Cleansing procedure removes source of the surface bacteria present around the urethral orifice.
• Perineum should be cleansed from front to back.	Prevents spreading bacteria from perirectal area to urethral orifice.
• Keeping labia separated, forcibly void a small amount (25 ml) into toilet.	The distal portion of the urethra contains bacteria. The forceful initial voiding will wash away these organisms. This minimizes the contamination of the urine from surface bacteria.
• Place *sterile* container *close to, but not touching,* the urethral orifice.	Sterile container is free from microorganisms that would contaminate the specimen and cause inaccurate findings from urine culture studies.

Key Steps	**Discussion**
• Void rest of urine into sterile container.	
Cap and label container.	Maintains sterility and identifies the person.

Male:

Instruct the man to do the following:

• Cleanse urethral orifice with sponge soaked in soap and water.	The noncircumcised male should pull back the foreskin and expose the orifice before washing.
• Forcibly void a small amount of urine (25 ml) into toilet.	
• Void all but the last few milliliters of urine into a sterile container.	
• Discard the last few milliliters of urine into toilet.	The final drops of urine contain prostatic secretions, which will contaminate the urine.
Cap and label container.	

Urine Testing for Glucose and Acetone

Two of the most commonly performed urine tests done by nurses are the tests for glucose and acetone.

Testing for glucose and acetone is frequently done for persons with known or suspected diabetes mellitus. To understand the purpose of these tests, you must review some of the mechanisms of renal physiology.

Ordinarily, all substances that are useful to the body are reabsorbed from the renal tubules before being excreted in the urine. Glucose is one of those substances that is reabsorbed completely. However, if the concentration of glucose in the blood is too high, the kidneys will not be able to reabsorb the entire amount of glucose before it is excreted in the urine. The point at which glucose begins to be lost through the tubules and into the urine is called the "renal threshold" for glucose (approximately 180 mg glucose/100 ml plasma).

In the person with diabetes, glucose is not able to be utilized by the cells. Glucose concentration in the blood rises and will appear in the urine if the renal threshold is exceeded. The greater the overload of glucose in the blood, the more glucose will appear in the urine.

The test for acetone (or ketones) in the urine indicates the amount of fat metabolism occurring in the body. Ketones are breakdown products of fatty acids and are produced in large numbers when the body breaks down large quantities of fats for energy. This process also occurs during diabetes. Because the body is not able to utilize glucose due to a deficiency of insulin, it begins to use fats as a source of energy. When ketones begin to appear in the urine, it is an indication that the body cells are severely deprived of needed glucose. This is always a serious sign for the person with diabetes.

Urine testing for the hospitalized person with diabetes is usually done before meals and at bedtime. This is because we need to know whether the glucose levels are elevated before the person ingests more carbohydrates at his next meal. If glucose is present in the urine, the physician may order a rapid-acting insulin to be given to "cover" the carbohydrate the person will ingest at the next meal. For this reason it is important to do the urine testing at the prescribed times and interpret the results accurately.

There are several commercially prepared products that are used for urine testing. The following procedure describes testing for glucose and acetone using Tes-Tape and Keto-Stix.

Procedure for Testing Urinary Glucose and Acetone (Using Tes-Tape and Keto-Stix)

Key Steps

Gather the following equipment:

- Urine specimen container
- Tes-Tape (measures glucose concentration)
- Keto-Stix (measures acetone concentration)

Give person specimen container. Instruct him to void. Save this specimen.

Instruct person to void again 30 minutes later. This is the specimen you will test.

Dip Tes-Tape into specimen.
Remove immediately. Tap against edge of specimen container.

Time the tape for 60 seconds, and read color change. (Time with your watch.) Tape will turn green in the presence of glucose.

Compare darkest area on tape to corresponding color on Tes-Tape container. Results are read as: negative, 1+, 2+, 3+, or 4+.

Repeat process with Keto-Stix. Time for 15 seconds before reading color change. Keto-Stix will turn purple in the presence of ketones.

Record time and results of test.

Discussion

Person may not be able to void again in 30 minutes, and you may need to test this first specimen.

Determines the person's current glucose level. The first voiding contains urine that was accumulated over several hours and may have a different glucose concentration than a recent specimen.

Removes excess urine.

Tape will continue to darken after 60 seconds and may give a false elevated reading. Tape changes colors because of a chemical reaction with glucose in the urine.

Darkest area gives most accurate index of glucose concentration.

Urine Specific Gravity

Specific gravity measures the weight of a given amount of solution compared to an equal amount of water. Because the weight of a solution depends on the number of dissolved particles it contains, specific gravity actually measures the concentration of dissolved particles in the solution. Solutions that are highly concentrated have high specific gravity readings. As the concentration of a solution becomes more dilute (contains more water and fewer particles) its specific gravity approaches 1.000.

Specific gravity is measured with an instrument called a hydrometer or urinometer. It consists of a mercury bulb attached to a stem with a graduated scale indicating a range of concentration from 1.000 to 1.040. The test is based on Archimedes' principle, which states that an object immersed in a solution displaces a certain amount of fluid. This object is "buoyed up" (or made to float) according to the weight of the fluid it displaces. When the hydrometer is placed in a concentrated solution, the weight of the fluid displaced is great, and the hydrometer is buoyed up and rises indicating a high specific gravity on the scale. When placed in less concentrated solution, the hydrometer displaces the same amount of fluid, but this fluid weighs less. There will be less buoyant force; the hydrometer will sink deeper into the solution, indicating a low specific gravity.

This test requires at least 20 ml of urine to give an accurate measurement. The normal range of specific gravity is approximately 1.010 to 1.025. This will vary from day to day and depends on several factors. For example, if there is a large loss of water, such as occurs in sweating, the specific gravity will increase.

Specific gravity is a useful index of renal function. The healthy kidney is able to concentrate urine according to the need of the body to retain or excrete fluids. When the kidney's ability to concentrate urine is impaired, active renal disease should be suspected. For example, the healthy kidneys will produce concentrated urine (with a high specific gravity) during dehydration when the body has an increased need to retain fluid. If you obtain a low specific gravity reading in the presence of dehydration, it would indicate that the kidneys were losing their ability to concentrate urine. This might be an early sign of impending renal failure.

Figure V-4 is a diagram of a hydrometer used to measure specific gravity. Each short line represents an increment of 0.001 on the scale. The long lines represent increments of 0.005 from the last long line. Read specific gravity from the bottom of the meniscus.

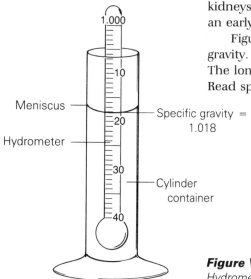

Figure V-4
Hydrometer measuring urine specific gravity

Procedure for Measuring Urine Specific Gravity

Key Steps   **Discussion**

Gather the following equipment:

  • Hydrometer with cylinder container

  • Urine specimen container

Key Steps	**Discussion**
Obtain a urine specimen from the person. (Must be at least 20 ml.)	Less than 20 ml will not provide adequate buoyant force to give an accurate reading.
Pour urine specimen into empty cylinder container.	
Place hydrometer into specimen by dipping it into the cylinder with a spinning motion.	Prevents hydrometer from leaning against the side of the container, which would give an inaccurate reading.
When urinometer stops spinning, read specific gravity at the bottom of the meniscus at eye level.	Most accurate reading is obtained at this level.
Record measurement and time.	

Enema Administration

Objectives

The student will be able to do the following:

1 Identify the proper position for administering an enema to a person.
2 Administer a soap suds enema and a commercially prepared enema.

Introduction

An enema is the introduction of fluid into the rectum and colon. The most common reason for giving rectal enemas is to stimulate peristalsis and the urge to defecate. The type of solution, amount, and frequency of administration is generally ordered by a physician.

There are several types of solution that may be prescribed, depending upon the purpose of the enema. The solution may be commercially prepared and come in disposable containers, or it may be prepared by the nurse before it is used. The most commonly used enemas are listed below.

- Tap water enema—a cleansing enema that distends the rectum, stimulating peristalsis. Usually 1000 ml of tap water is used.

- Soap suds enema—a cleansing enema that by chemical irritation distends and stimulates the colon. Usually one package of castile soap to 1000 ml of tap water is used.

- Mineral oil (retention) enema—a softening enema that lubricates the lining of the bowel as well as stool. It can also stimulate peristalsis by volume. Usually 150 ml to 200 ml of mineral oil, cottonseed oil, or olive oil is used.

- Commercially prepared cleansing enema—a cleansing enema consisting of a hypertonic solution that causes distention by creating a fluid bulk in the colon from osmosis of body fuids. It also acts as a mild irritant on the bowel mucosa. It usually comes in a 4-ounce enema unit.

The principles and rationale for administration of enemas are generally the same with all of the solutions. The procedure for administration of a soap suds enema is described here, followed by modifications for commercial types of cleansing enemas and retention enemas.

Procedure for Administering a Soap Suds Enema

Key Steps	*Discussion*
Collect the following equipment: • Water soluble lubricant • Blue pad • Bedpan • Portable IV pole • Enema bag • Liquid castile soap	
Fill enema bag with warm water. Temperature of solution should be near 105° F. This should feel warm on wrist. Hand bag from IV pole. Add liquid soap.	Warm water will not be harmful to the mucous membrane lining of the colon and rectum. Vasoconstriction and cramping can occur with water that is too cold. Burning can occur with hot water.
Open the clamp and allow the solution to run through the tubing to expel the air.	Instillation of air into colon can cause flatus, cramping, and shorter retention time.
Approach and identify the person. Explain procedure and purpose.	Minimizes anxiety.
Prepare the person as follows: • Provide for privacy. • Position the patient on his left side. • Place blue pad under buttocks.	Ensures patient comfort. The enema solution flows through the rectum and sigmoid colon to the descending colon more easily.
Lubricate 4 inches to 6 inches of tubing.	Promotes easier passage of tube.
Ask the person to take deep breaths through his mouth.	Helps to relax the anal and rectal muscles.
Insert the lubricated rectal tube slowly and gently about 4 inches.	The rectum of an adult person is approximately 7 inches to 8 inches in length.

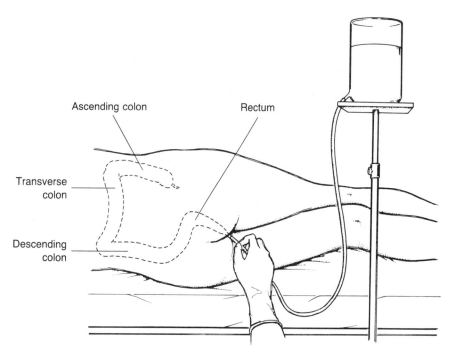

Key Steps

Open clamp, and instill the solution slowly into the bowel. Hold the solution container 12 inches to 18 inches above the anus.

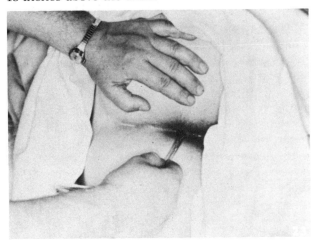

Discussion

Regulate the flow according to the person's ability to retain it for comfort and to avoid damage to the mucous membranes. At 12 inches to 18 inches the solution will enter the bowel but will not cause undue pressure and dilitation.

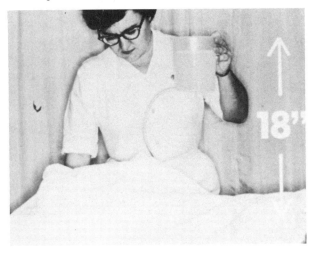

Pinch the tubing, and remove the rectal tube when all solution is instilled or patient is unable to hold any more.

Assist person to bathroom or place on the bedpan.

Discard all equipment.

Chart results and person's tolerance to the procedure.

Prevents air from entering the tube and leakage of solution onto bed.

Better results are achieved with person in a natural sitting position unless contraindicated by his condition.

Note color, amount, and consistency of stool.

Modifications

If using a commercially prepared enema, warm it in a basin of water or under a warm tap. Lubricate the tip and insert it into the rectum. Compress the enema until all the solution has been administered.

If a retention enema is administered, encourage the person to hold the enema until it is absorbed or for the amount of time indicated to achieve the desired therapeutic effect.

Bowel Diversion

Objectives

The student will be able to do the following:

1 Perform a colostomy irrigation.
2 Apply a new drainage bag to a stoma.
3 State rationale for meticulous skin care for persons with bowel diversions.

Introduction

A bowel diversion creates an artificial opening from the bowel through the abdomen through which fecal material exits. A colostomy involves the large intestine, usually the transverse, descending, or sigmoid colon. An ileostomy involves the ileum or terminal portion of the small intestine. A pouch is worn over the stoma, or opening, to collect bowel contents. Bowel diversions create obvious alterations in body image as well as in physical function. While performing physical care, nurses are sensitive to the person's emotional adjustment and needs. Teaching self-care is an important intervention to assist these persons to achieve a sense of control.

Because bowel contents are irritating to the skin, meticulous care is necessary to prevent skin breakdown. This care is especially important for persons with ileostomies because bowel contents contain more digestive enzymes with ileostomies than with colostomies. Odor control is another concern for individuals with bowel diversions. Finally, the person with a colostomy may need to learn how to perform periodic irrigations, a procedure which flushes out fecal material (much like an enema) and may help to develop bowel control. Procedures for changing an ostomy appliance and doing skin care, and a method of colostomy irrigation are described below.

Procedure for Stoma Care

Key Steps

Discussion

Assemble the following equipment:
- Blue pad
- Bedpan
- Skin barrier (Stomahesive, karaya sheets, and karaya powder are common types)
- Soap and water
- Irrigating syringe
- New drainage bag (if needed)
- Scissors
- Protective spray or lotion (such as tincture of benzoin)

Explain procedure to the person.

Gains cooperation and participation, and allays anxiety.

Assist person to a supine position, and screen for privacy.

Expose only the working area, and protect the bed with a blue pad.

Wash your hands.

Promotes cleanliness, and prevents infection.

If bag is not to be removed:
Open bottom of bag for drainage of fecal material (measure). Irrigate bag with warm soapy water using irrigating syringe. Hold end of bag shut and swish solution around inside bag for thorough cleansing.

Maintains cleanliness, and prevents unpleasant odors.

Drain and instill clear water for rinsing. Drain off water. Close bag, folding the end two or three times, and apply binder clip. Go on to last step of the procedure for stoma care.

Key Steps

Discussion

If bag is to be removed:
Change bags when they leak, become odorous, or skin irritation develops.

Remove bag, and cleanse area around stoma. Wash gently and thoroughly with soap and water. Pat thoroughly dry.

Prevents skin breakdown from decomposed fecal material by keeping area clean and dry.

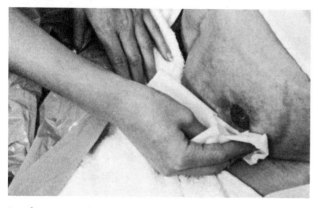

Apply protective spray or liquid (if indicated).

Prevents skin irritation from exposure to fecal material.

Measure the stoma (measuring guides are usually available). Hole in skin barrier should fit exactly around stoma. Hole in the drainage bag should leave no more than ⅛-inch margin exposed around stoma. Cut hole in skin barrier, remove backing, and apply over stoma. Remove backing from drainage bag to expose adhesive surface, and apply over skin barrier, centering hole in drainage bag over the stoma. In order to obtain a complete seal, first apply pressure to seal the part of the bag that is proximal to the opening, then seal the remaining part smoothly to the skin barrier.

Close-fitting appliance prevents fecal material from contacting skin.

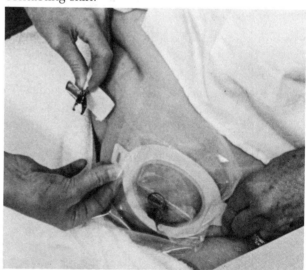

Close the bag, folding the end two or three times, and apply binder clip.

Adjust strap or belt, if person has either, to make sure bag is held in place.

Clean up equipment, and provide for the person's comfort.

Chart pertinent observations such as condition of skin, client teaching, and appearance of stool.

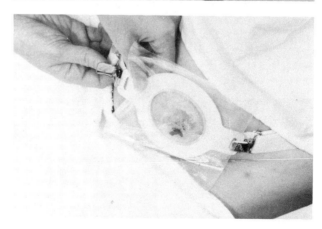

Procedure for Irrigating a Colostomy

Key Steps

Gather the following equipment:

- Irrigating bag (open-ended colostomy bag)
- Enema bag
- Irrigation solution
- Lubricant
- IV pole
- Colostomy bag
- Skin barrier
- Protective spray (if desired)
- Scissors

Prepare a liter of solution, and warm it to 105° F. Pour into enema bag. If thermometer is not available, you may test the temperature of tap water by running the water over the inner surface of your wrist. It should be warm, not hot. Hang enema bag from IV pole.

Explain procedure to the person.

Position person in bed on his side. Place blue pads on the bed under the person's side. If irrigation is done in the bathroom, assist the person to sit on the commode.

Remove colostomy bag and dispose of it.

Position open-ended colostomy bag over stoma. Be sure to put end of bag into bedpan (or toilet) to direct the flow.

Expel the air from the tubing of enema bag before insertion by allowing fluid to run through.

Lubricate the distal 3 inches to 4 inches of the tubing.

Discussion

Solution that is too cold can cause vasoconstriction and cramping. If solution is too hot, it may cause a thermal injury.

Helps to prevent or allay anxiety, and promotes cooperation.

Makes stomal area accessible.

Failure to release air from tubing before inserting will increase flatus and may cause cramping.

Promotes ease of insertion.

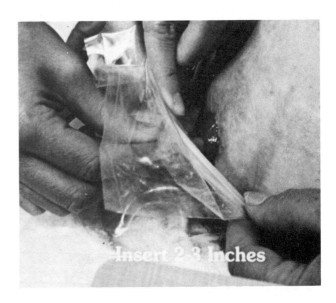

Key Steps	*Discussion*

The height of bag should be no more than 12 inches to 18 inches when person is in bed, at shoulder level when person is in bathroom.

The rate of flow of a solution varies with the pressure gradient, caliber of the tube, and density of the fluid. Flow will flow only where there is a difference in pressure between solution in the container and the end of the outflow tube. If pressure is too great, muscles of the intestinal walls contract too quickly and cause much pain.

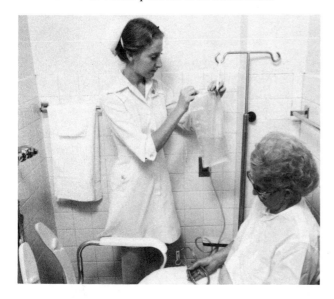

Insert the tube *slowly* and gently 3 inches to 4 inches—rotate catheter as you insert. It may go in easier if you unclamp the tube and allow fluid to flow. Remember, if there is difficulty inserting the tubing, withdraw it and reinsert. *Never force.*

Difficulty inserting the catheter may be caused by a hard piece of stool or obstruction. Forcing the catheter may traumatize the mucous membrane or perforate the colon.

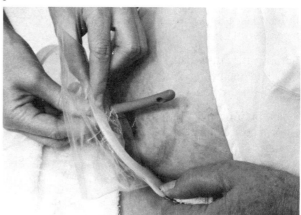

Run in about 250 ml to 500 ml of solution at a time, depending on person's ability to retain it. If the person complains of cramping, pinch the tubing and have person take deep breaths through the mouth and relax; then continue the flow. If cramps continue, lower the irrigating can.

Allow solution to drain out of bowel.

Sufficient solution is needed to start peristaltic action, but too much solution will cause excessive distention of part to be irrigated. Slight cramping may simply be a signal that the bowel is ready to empty. Severe cramping is caused by solution that is too cold or by excessive pressure.

Fluid return is caused by peristalsis. The flow into the bag is caused by the force of gravity (high level to low level).

Key Steps

Failure of fluid to return may occur occasionally. To encourage the return, one or more of the following steps may be taken:

- Gentle massage of lower abdomen
- Tightening the abdominal muscles
- Taking several deep breaths and relaxing
- Gently twisting the body (at waist) from side to side
- Standing up or sitting more erect

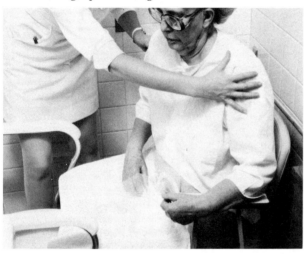

Repeat last four steps until return flow is clear of feces and flatus.

Remove irrigating bag. Cleanse stoma, and apply new bag according to procedure for stoma care described previously.

Chart time of irrigation, results, person's reaction to procedure, and any change in his condition such as extreme weakness, dizziness, or pain.

Discussion

This may be caused by the catheter being inserted too far, or water can be trapped behind a hard stool and may be absorbed.

Removal of all fecal matter at this time may prevent drainage of fecal material later on in the day.

Prevents skin irritation and maceration.

Fluid and Electrolytes

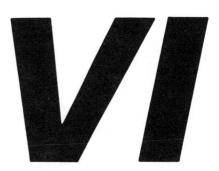

Maintenance of fluid and electrolyte balance is one important factor determining health. In health, many mechanisms operate to balance gains and losses of water and electrolytes, including renal functions and hormones such as antidiuretic hormone (ADH) or aldosterone. In illness, however, regulatory mechanisms are often disrupted, causing imbalances in body chemistry.

Monitoring fluid intake and output is one means by which nurses can assess persons with potential fluid imbalances. Accurate measurement of fluid gain or loss is often the basis for determining appropriate interventions. This section describes the procedure for measuring fluid intake and output.

Intravenous therapy is often employed when fluid or electrolyte imbalances exist. A discussion of techniques related to intravenous therapy can be found in Section X of this manual.

Intake and Output Measurement

Objectives

The student will be able to do the following:

1 State indications for measuring intake and output.

2 Describe the procedure for measuring and recording intake and output.

Introduction

Measuring a person's fluid intake and output is a very important part of estimating the state of fluid balance. In health, the body maintains several regulating mechanisms so that water intake is balanced against water loss. In illness, intake may exceed output or vice versa and may result in a serious state of fluid imbalance if undetected and untreated. An accurate measurement of fluid intake and output (I and O) can inform health-care providers whether fluid balance is being maintained.

Nurses do not need a physician's order to measure I and O but can and should record it for any person who may have a fluid balance problem. Conditions in which I and O should be recorded include the following:

- NPO for longer than 24 hours
- Immediate postoperative period
- Prolonged fever
- Bleeding
- Fluid loss through drainage tubes, burns, or prolonged vomiting or diarrhea
- Fluid overload or dehydration

Measuring Fluid Intake

Fluid intake occurs through the following routes:

- Oral
- Feeding tubes
- Intravenous infusions

Fluid intake is measured and recorded using the metric system. All fluid is recorded in milliliters (ml). The route of fluid intake is also recorded (e.g., oral, tube feeding, intravenous infusion). Most institutions have standard forms for recording I and O at the bedside or in the client's record.

Fluid is also gained from solid food and through metabolic processes. These routes are not considered in the written intake record, however. Solid food is not included in I and O measurements.

Oral Fluid Intake

To check oral intake, note the liquids the person has consumed and how much of each. For example:

½ carton of milk

1 cup of coffee

1 5-oz cup of juice

Most institutions provide a list of fluid equivalents of their standard dietary containers. If the client is maintaining an intake record at home, he may need assistance to standardize the containers used for measuring intake. Convert the amount of liquid consumed to milliliters, and calculate the total intake.

Feeding Tube Intake

Tube feedings are liquids that are administered through a tube that is placed in the gastrointestinal tract. All fluids administered through the tube are recorded in milliliters on the I and O slip at the time of each feeding, and the route is noted.

Intravenous Intake

Intravenous intake is recorded in milliliters on the I and O slip, and the route is noted. Intravenous intake is usually recorded each time a container is infused and at the end of each shift. If a container of intravenous solution is only partially infused, note the amount of solution left in the container, and subtract from the total amount of solution present when the container was hung.

Measuring Fluid Output

Fluid output is produced by the following:

- Urine
- Feces
- Perspiration
- Respiration
- Abnormal losses (vomiting, diarrhea, bleeding, drainage tubes)

Fluid that is lost through feces, perspiration, or respiration is not usually included on a written I and O record. If the person is losing a large amount of fluid through abnormal respiration or profuse perspiration, this is charted in the nurse's notes. In such instances, weighing the client may give the best indication of fluid loss. Liquid stools or diarrhea are usually measured and included in written I and O records.

Procedure for Measuring Intake and Output

Key Steps

Discussion

Intake:
Inform client of procedure and purpose.

Elicits participation in accurate measurement of intake.

Key Steps

Check meal tray's containers, and record liquids consumed.

Convert the amount of liquids consumed to milliliters, calculate total intake, and list under intake column of I and O slip. Note route (*e.g.,* oral) (Fig. VI-1).

Intake and Output Chart
Days 8 a.m.–4 p.m.

Name .... *John Smith* ....

Date ..... *3/31* .... Bed No. ....

Hour		Intake	Output	
			Urinary	Nonurinary
8:00	Good Fair Poor			
9:00		*100 PO*	*350*	
10:00				
11:00				
12:00	Good Fair Poor	*150 PO*	*500*	
1:00				
2:00			*150*	
3:00		*1000 ml–IV*		*300–N.G.*
Total		*1150*	*1000*	*300*

University of Michigan—University Hospital

H-2060322

Record other oral liquid intake appropriately.

Record amount of tube feedings in milliliters on I and O slip, and note route.

Record intravenous fluids on I and O slip, and note route.

Output:
Ask client to save all urine for measurement.

Pour urine into graduated container, note amount of milliliters, and record under output column of I and O slip. Note route.

Measure nonurinary output such as liquid stools, drainage from tubes, and vomitus. Use a graduated container, obtain the amount in milliliters, and record as nonurinary output.

Discussion

Example:
½ carton of milk
1 cup of coffee

Example:
½ carton of milk	= 120 ml
1 cup of coffee	= 140 ml
	260 ml

Figure VI-1
Intake and output record

Example: water at the bedside, ice cream, juice

Elicits participation in accurate measurement of output.

Note the source of output (*e.g.,* gastric drainage, ileostomy).

Circulation

VII

Every person experiences stressors that affect the cardiovascular system. In some instances these factors may seriously disrupt oxygen supply to cells. With the following procedures, students will learn skills to help them assess the function of the person's circulatory system and intervene for selected problems. Included in this section are skills related to vital signs, assessment of peripheral pulses, and application of elastic bandages and stockings.

Vital Signs

Objectives

The student will be able to do the following:

1 Take vital signs accurately.
2 Auscultate the apical pulse.
3 Take an apical–radial pulse.

Introduction

Vital signs are parameters of body function that reveal a person's state of health. The cardinal or vital signs include body temperature, pulse, respirations, and blood pressure. Because vital signs are usually assessed together, all four are described in this section.

Measurement of Body Temperature

Body temperature is a measure of the balance of heat production and heat loss of the body. Multiple factors affect temperature maintenance and regulation, including external environment (room temperature, ventilation, clothing), internal environment (amount of adipose tissue, illness, state of hydration), age, time of day, menstrual cycle, emotional status, activity, and drugs.

Under normal conditions, the body temperature remains in a fairly constant range as a result of the control exercised by the heat-regulating center located in the hypothalamus of the brain. "Fever" exists when heat regulation is not keeping pace with heat production or the body is producing heat at a faster rate than the hypothalamus can control.

Glass Thermometer

The typical thermometer used to measure body temperature is glass and contains mercury, a metal which readily expands when it is exposed to heat. It registers temperature in units called degrees, and it is usually marked according to the Fahrenheit scale. The other temperature scale is called Celsius or centigrade. On the Fahrenheit scale, the range for normal body temperature is considered to be between 97°F (36°C) and 99°F (37.2°C) to account for individual variations. A reading of 99°F or above is considered a significant elevation.

Figure VII-1 is a diagram of the Fahrenheit scale on a glass thermometer. On this scale, the longer lines represent one degree (1°) of temperture, and each small line represents two tenths (0.2°) of a degree.

Body temperature is usually measured in the mouth, rectum, or axilla. Traditionally, rectal temperatures have been considered to be

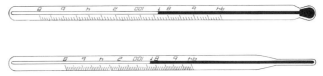

Figure VII-1

Clinical thermometers used for measuring body temperature. The upper thermometer is used to record mouth temperatures. The thermometer at the bottom is used for rectal temperatures. Note that the column of mercury is at 98.6°F in both thermometers. All clinical thermometers sold in the United States soon will be marked with both Fahrenheit and Celsius scales.

1°F higher and axillary temperatures 1°F lower than oral temperature recordings. However, this has not been documented by research, and we can only assume that rectal readings are the highest and axillary readings the lowest.[1] Regardless of the site chosen, the bulb or tip of the thermometer must be placed so that it is surrounded by body tissue with a good blood supply and in as closed a space as possible. The nurse determines the route by which a temperature will be taken after considering factors such as age, level of consciousness, diagnosis, and the ability of the person to breathe through the nose during the procedure.

Every unit and hospital has its own method for thermometer sterilization, but the thermometer must always be disinfected after use to prevent the spread of microorganisms. Thermometers may be rinsed under cool water but never under hot water because heat causes mercury to expand, and the thermometer may break.

Procedure for Measuring Oral Temperature with Glass Thermometer

Key Steps

Discussion

Wash hands.

Prevents spread of microorganisms.

Gather the following equipment:

- Oral thermometer (glass)
- Tissue
- Paper
- Pencil

Pick up the thermometer by the stem (not bulb).

Avoids contamination of the thermometer.

Grasp the thermometer with the thumb and first two fingers, raise the thermometer in a horizontal position to eye level, and rotate slowly until the column of mercury is clearly visible against the calibrations.

Check for the following:

- Any crack or chips
- Worn number or indistinct calibrations
- Split mercury column
- Full reservoir of mercury in the bulb

Read the height of mercury column by comparing it to the numbered calibrations on the thermometer. If necessary, prepare to shake the mercury down in the thermometer as follows:

Because of the constriction just above the bulb of the thermometer that keeps the mercury from falling, it may be necessary to shake the mercury down to well below the normal temperature level to achieve an accurate reading.

- Lower the thermometer, and position yourself so that you cannot strike the thermometer against an object.

Avoids breaking the thermometer.

Key Steps

Discussion

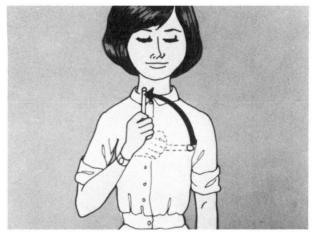

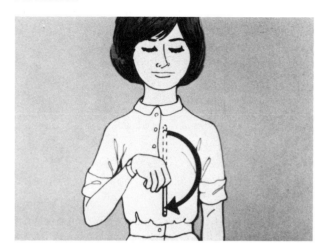

- Keeping the wrist loose, raise the wrist slightly and flick it downward in a sharp whip-cracking motion three or four times.

Again, raise the thermometer to eye level and recheck the height of the column of mercury.

Continue the shaking-down procedure until the mercury is at a point well below the normal temperature level, at least to 96° or less.

Instruct the person to open his mouth slightly and raise his tongue.

Place the thermometer under the tongue at a 45° angle. Locate the thermometer at posterior base of tongue.

This is the position that allows the bulb to rest against the tongue tissue comfortably and that records highest oral temperature reading. Incorrect placement at the anterior tongue results in a lower, incorrect reading.

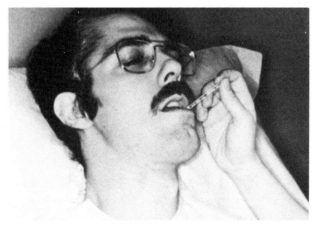

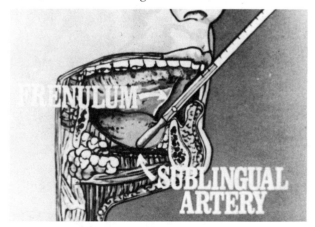

With the thermometer resting on the person's lower lip, request him to lower his tongue until the bulb is completely covered.

Instruct the person to close his mouth carefully with the lips held firmly together and not to bite down on the thermometer with his teeth.

Maintains a closed internal cavity.

Leave the thermometer in place for 8 minutes.

Time needed for correct oral temperature to record on thermometer.[2]

Key Steps

Discussion

Grasp the thermometer stem, request the person to open his mouth, and gently remove the thermometer from under the tongue.

Take a tissue and wipe the thermometer.

Cleanse thermometer of any secretions to facilitate reading.

Raise the thermometer to eye level, rotate it slowly to locate the mercury column, and read the height of the column.

Record the reading immediately on a piece of paper so that it will not be forgotten.

Again, position yourself away from any objects, and shake down the thermometer.

Place the thermometer in the container labeled "dirty."

The thermometers will all be cleansed at the same time and returned to the clean container.

Wash your hands.

Chart the temperature reading, time and date obtained, and related observations such as diaphoresis.

Procedure for Measuring Rectal Temperature

Key Steps

Discussion

Same as previously outlined with the following modifications:
Position person on his side with knees slightly flexed.

This position provides a clear view of the external anal sphincter muscle of the rectum.

Fold back the covers carefully so that there is no undue exposure of the person.

Apply water-soluble lubricant to the bulb end of the thermometer to a level of approximately 1 inch above the bulb (a total of approximately 1½ inches).

With the thumb and index fingers of one hand, gently separate the buttocks until the anus can clearly be seen.

Insert the lubricated thermometer bulb into the rectum for approximately 1½ inches.

The rectal bulb should be inserted into the rectum so that it rests just past the anal canal, which is approximately 1 inch in length.

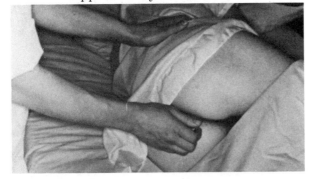

Key Steps

Permit the buttocks to fall back into place.

Leave the thermometer in place for 2 minutes to 3 minutes, holding onto it with your fingers. Remain with the person.

Discussion

Prevents injury to person, and obtains an accurate reading.[2]

Procedure for Measuring Axillary Temperature

Key Steps

Same as outlined for oral temperature with the following modifications:
Position person in a comfortable position.

Place the thermometer in the axillary region with the bulb in the center of the axilla, where the highest axillary temperature can be obtained.

Discussion

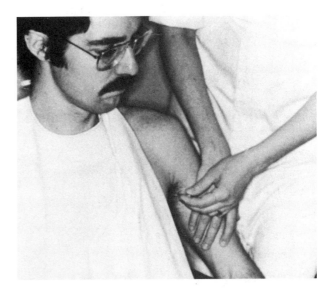

Place the person's arm across his chest and hold the arm securely in place in order to hold the thermometer in place.

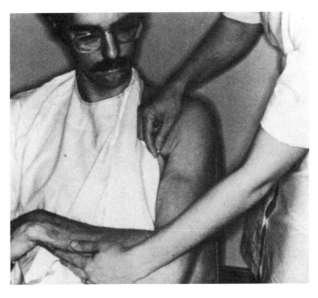

Leave the thermometer in place for 9 minutes.

Time required for accurate reading.[3]

Electronic Thermometer

Many hospitals now use an electronic instrument to monitor body temperature. Some of the advantages offered by electronic thermometers are the following:

- Temperature readings can be obtained within approximately 20 seconds
- Readings are accurate to within plus or minus two tenths of 1 degree
- The hazard of accidental glass breakage is eliminated
- Disposable probe covers prevent cross contamination

Accurate oral temperatures can be obtained on many persons who mouth breathe, intubated and comatose persons, and small children who would have needed rectal temperatures if a glass thermometer were used.

In general, electronic thermometers consist of the following components: the temperature-taking unit, which the nurse carries to the person's bedside; removable probes, one type for oral and axillary temperatures, another for rectal temperatures; the battery charger, which also serves as the storage stand for the electronic thermometer when it is not in use; and the disposable plastic probe covers.

Procedure for Taking Oral Temperature with Electronic Thermometer

Key Steps

Wash hands.

Gather the following equipment:

- Electronic thermometer
- Disposable probe covers
- Paper
- Pencil

Discussion

Prevents spread of microorganisms.

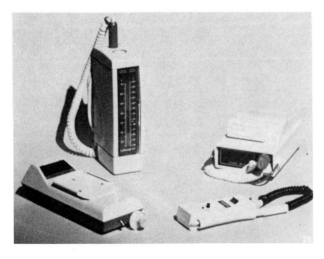

Be sure that oral probe is connected to unit.

Insert probe firmly into plastic probe cover. Do not touch probe cover with your hands.

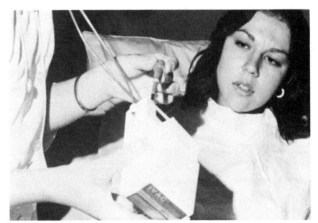

Prevents possible contamination.

Key Steps

Discussion

Instruct person to open his mouth slightly and raise his tongue.

Place the probe under the tongue with the tip resting at the posterior base of the tongue to record highest oral temperature.

Instruct the person to lower his tongue until probe tip is covered and to close his mouth.

Maintains a closed cavity.

Hold probe in position until the signal appears indicating temperature has been recorded. The temperature reading will be displayed on electronic unit.

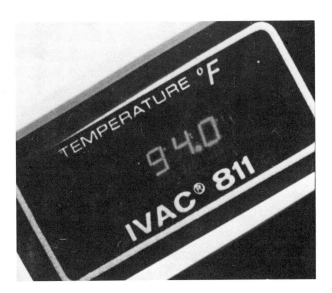

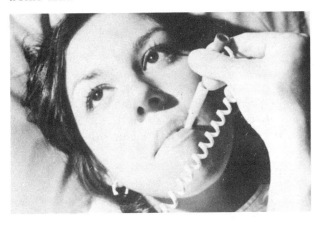

Ask person to open mouth; remove probe.

Hold probe over waste container and release probe cover by pushing on end of probe with finger. Eject probe cover directly into waste container. This avoids contaminating hands with saliva.

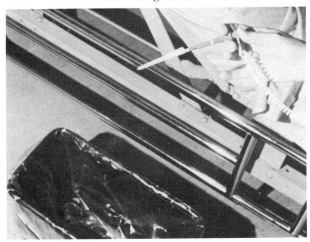

Return probe to holder.

Resets unit for next reading, and protects probe.

Chart the reading, time and date obtained, and related observations such as diaphoresis.

Modifications

For axillary temperature, use the oral probe, and follow the procedure just outlined with modifications in Procedure for Measuring Axillary Temperature, p 123. For rectal temperature, use the rectal probe, and follow the procedure just outlined with modifications in Procedure for Measuring Rectal Temperature, p 122.

Measurement of Pulse

Pulse represents the beat of the heart as felt through the walls of the arteries—a shock wave that travels along the fibers of the arteries as the heart contracts. Three determinants of arterial pulse are the following:

- Blood volume (blood supply)
- Cardiac output (force of contraction of the left ventricle)
- Elasticity (a resistance or tension) of the arterial walls or blood vessels

  Factors that affect the pulse rate are:

- Physical activity
- Age (The pulse rate of a child is higher than that of an adult. The pulse rate of the elderly person is higher than that of an adult because the elderly have more rigid arteries, which increase the work of the heart.)
- Emotional stress or pain
- Ingesting a heavy meal
- Smoking

Because so many factors affect the pulse rate, there is not a specific "normal" rate for all individuals. However, the usual range for an adult in a resting state is above 60 beats per minute and below 100 beats per minute. Pulses are also assessed for rhythm and quality or volume. A normal pulse is regular, with an equal interval between each beat, and is easily palpated.

In order to palpate the muscular walls of the arteries, it is necessary that they be close to the skin surface and lying over a firm structure. The pulse is most commonly taken at the inner aspect or thumb side of the wrist because here the radial artery lies over bone and is near the surface of the body. Other common sites to palpate or feel the pulse are over the temporal artery in front of the ear and slightly above the level of the eye and at the carotid artery on the lateral aspect of the neck. When measuring a pulse by palpation, place two or three fingers over the pulse site, and gently press. Never feel a pulse with your thumb, because it has a pulse of its own which may interfere with an accurate measurement.

Another way to measure the pulse is to listen to the heartbeat with a stethoscope at the apex of the heart. This method is known as taking the pulse by auscultation as opposed to taking the pulse by palpation. The apex is the lower blunt tip of the heart mass, approximately two thirds of which lies to the left of the midline of the anterior chest. The apical pulse is the sound produced by the closure of the atrial-ventricular and semi-lunar valves during the cardiac cycle. An apical pulse determination results in the most accurate determination of rate.

Occasionally, the apical and radial pulses are assessed simultaneously to determine whether a pulse deficit exists. Pulse deficit is the difference between radial and apical pulse rates and reflects inefficient ventricular contractions that eject no blood. Such contractions produce heart sounds but no palpable pulse wave. Pulse deficits may be found in persons experiencing atrial fibrillation or premature ventricular contractions.

Procedure for Measuring Radial Pulse

Key Steps	*Discussion*
Wash your hands.	Prevents cross contamination.
Gather the following equipment: • Watch with second hand • Paper • Pencil	
Position the person's arm in a natural alignment with the body.	If the person is in a sitting position, rest the arm on the bed or bedside table so that it is relaxed and on a level with the heart. If the person is lying down, place the arm in a relaxed position alongside of the body. Never raise the arm above the level of the heart because this causes the flow of blood to oppose the pull of gravity and, as a result, the pulse rate will rise.
Turn the palm of the person's hand downward.	This position places the radial artery in its natural position on the inner aspect (thumb side) of the person's wrist.

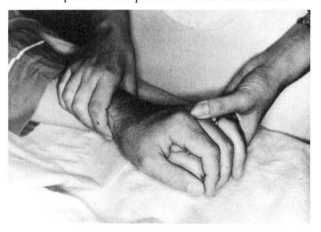

Gently place the first two or three fingers of your hand on the person's radial artery and press the artery against the bone until the pulse is palpated. Rest your thumb on the back of the person's wrist.	The person's pulse is not felt with your thumb because it has its own pulse. Gentle pressure is applied so as not to completely obliterate the artery.
Keep your fingers gently on the pulse and count the number of pulsations for 15 seconds. Note the rhythm and volume also.	Multiply the rate for 15 seconds by 4 to get the rate for a full minute.
Immediately record the rate, rhythm, and volume of the pulse on a piece of paper.	Prevents possible error caused by delayed recording from memory.
Chart the rate, any alterations in rhythm and volume, date and time obtained, and related observations.	

Procedure for Measuring Apical Pulse

Key Steps	Discussion
Wash hands.	Prevents cross contamination.
Gather the following equipment: • Watch with second hand • Stethoscope • Alcohol sponge • Paper • Pencil	
Clean earpieces of stethoscope with alcohol.	Prevents spread of microorganisms by way of earpieces.
Position the person comfortably either lying or sitting in bed or seated in a chair. If the patient is in a sitting position, request him to lean slightly forward.	The forward position increases the contact of the apex of the heart against the chest wall and makes it easier to hear the apical beat through the stethoscope.
Screen the person for privacy.	
Open the person's gown, shirt or blouse, and without undue exposure, bare the left chest.	Clothing interferes with accurate auscultation.
Locate the apex of the heart by placing your finger in the center of the left clavicle and drawing an imaginary line down the chest to a point just under the nipple of the left breast.	This point should correspond with the apex of the heart, which is located between the fifth and sixth ribs in the fifth intercostal space of the left anterior chest.
Place the earpieces of the stethoscope in a forward position in your ear canals.	This position follows the normal anatomical position of the ear canals.
Place the diaphragm or bell of the stethoscope over the apex of the heart in a manner that does not unduly expose the patient.	

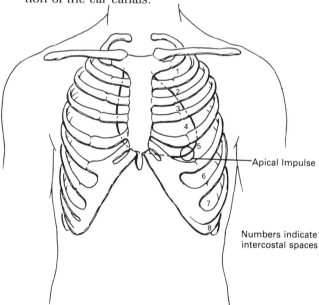

Apical Impulse

Numbers indicate intercostal spaces

Count the number of beats for 1 minute. Note also the rhythm and volume.	You will hear two sounds that together equal one beat.

Key Steps	*Discussion*
Remove the stethoscope, and replace the person's clothing.	
Immediately record the rate, rhythm, and volume of the apical pulse on a piece of paper.	
Cleanse the earpieces of the stethoscope with an alcohol sponge.	When the stethoscope is used by more than one person, it should be cleansed with an alcohol sponge between use to prevent the spread of microorganisms.
Chart the rate, any alterations in rhythm or volume, date and time obtained, and related observations.	

Procedure for Determining Apical–Radial Pulse Rate

Key Steps	*Discussion*
One nurse places the stethoscope over the apex of the heart. A second nurse places his or her fingers on the radial pulse. The nurse who is counting the apical pulse acts as the timer and marks by some prearranged signal when the simultaneous counting of the apical–radial rates should begin and when they should stop.	A simultaneous count assures the most accurate determination of differences in apical and radial rates.
Both nurses then record their readings and determine the pulse deficit.	

Measurement of Respirations

Measurement of respiration means noting the number of respiratory cycles (consisting of an inspiratory and expiratory phase) per minute. Because of the close relationship between the pulmonary and cardiovascular systems, the same factors that affect the pulse affect respirations. Because so many factors affect respirations, there is no one normal rate for all individuals. A normal range is approximately 12 respirations to 20 respirations per minute.

When observing a person's respirations, note the depth and rhythm of the respirations as well as the rate. Rhythm measures the regularity and evenness of respirations. Depth represents an estimate of the amount of volume of air that is exchanged in each respiration. Therefore, in recording respirations it might be noted that a person's respiratory rate is 20 per minute and the respirations are regular and of adequate or normal depth. On the other hand, it might be noted that the person's respiratory rate is 40 per minute and the respirations are irregular and shallow.

Procedure for Measuring Respirations

Key Steps	*Discussion*

Equipment is same as that for pulse determination as follows:

- Watch with second hand
- Paper
- Pencil

After counting the radial pulse rate, continue to hold your fingers on the pulse for another full minute so that the rate, depth, and rhythm of respirations can be counted unobtrusively.

Because respirations are to an extent under voluntary control, accuracy is best achieved if the person is not overly aware of the counting of his respirations. If respirations are difficult to observe, place the person's arm across his chest. Leaving your fingers on the radial pulse while counting the respirations you will be able to feel the rise and fall of the chest with each inspiration and expiration.

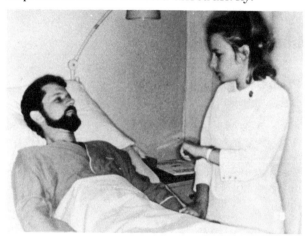

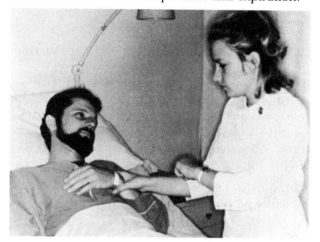

Immediately record the rate, rhythm, and volume of the respirations on a piece of paper.

Chart the rate, any alterations in volume and rhythm, and date and time obtained.

Measurement of Blood Pressure

Blood pressure is the measurement of the force of blood against the walls of the arteries. Blood pressure is measured in millimeters of mercury (mm Hg), which represents the height to which a column of mercury would rise were it exposed to the force of arterial circulation. Blood pressure is the product of two forces, cardiac output and peripheral resistance. There are two components to a blood pressure reading: systolic pressure, which represents cardiac contraction and chiefly reflects cardiac output, and diastolic pressure, which represents ventricular filling and chiefly reflects peripheral resistance. Normal systolic pressure ranges from 90 mm Hg to 130 mm Hg; diastolic pressure normally ranges from 60 mm Hg to 90 mm Hg. Anxiety, fear, food ingestion, exercise, and age all are associated with an increase in blood pressure.

Blood pressure is commonly measured by an instrument called a sphygmomanometer, which consists of a rubber bladder inside of a cloth cuff, a pressure bulb with a control valve that is attached to the cuff by tubing, and a pressure gauge. In order to obtain accurate readings, the bladder length should encompass one half of the person's arm circumference, and the cuff width should be approximately 40% of the arm circumference. Use of a too-narrow cuff provides falsely high pressures, while a cuff that is too wide results in falsely low readings. The cuff should be wrapped snugly because loose application causes falsely high readings. Bulky dressings or clothing under cuffs also cause falsely high readings.[4]

When auscultating blood pressure sounds, note three points recommended by the American Heart Association: the level at which sounds first appear (systolic pressure), the level at which sounds muffle (first diastolic pressure), and the level at which sounds disappear (second diastolic pressure). A blood pressure reading obtained in this manner might be written as 120/80/70. Yet, in common practice only the systolic and second diastolic pressures are noted. This can be problematic in persons whose sounds can be heard all the way to the zero level on the sphygmomanometer. In this case the point of muffling is commonly recorded as the diastolic blood pressure. Obviously, common clinical practice allows confusion as to how a blood pressure reading was determined. It is best to note all three sounds when recording blood pressure or to determine whether there is a standard institutional procedure for blood pressure measurement and follow recommendations.

Procedure for Measuring Blood Pressure

Key Steps

Wash hands.

Gather the following equipment:
- Sphygmomanometer with cuff
- Stethoscope
- Alcohol sponge
- Paper
- Pencil

Explain procedure to the person. Use measures to alleviate anxiety if necessary.

Open the control valve on the pressure bulb completely.

Roll up the cuff and squeeze it between both hands, or place on firm surface with cuff open to full length and press firmly.

Discussion

Prevents spread of microorganisms.

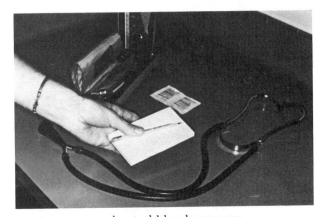

Anxiety causes elevated blood pressure.

Compress cuff to release all trapped air in the rubber bag.

Key Steps

Roll the person's sleeve well above the bend on the elbow. If the sleeve of the garment cannot be rolled with ease or is constricting when rolled, take the arm out of the sleeve.

Place the person's arm in the appropriate position as follows:

- Heart level
- Extended at full length
- Palm turned upward
- Inner aspect of the arm exposed
- Well supported and relaxed

Place the cuff over the person's upper arm so that the inflatable rubber bag inside the cuff is centered over the brachial artery and the lower edge of the cuff is approximately 1 inch above the antecubital fossa (the bend of the elbow).

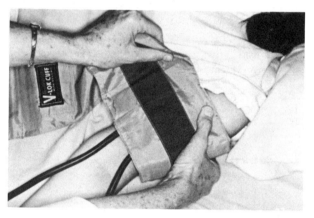

Wrap the cuff smoothly, evenly, and snugly around the person's upper arm. Lock the Velcro surfaces so that the cuff is secure, or tuck in the end of a cloth cuff securely.

Face the manometer scale, which should be placed in a vertical position on a flat surface. You should be no further than 3 feet from the scale, and your eye should be level with the mercury column. An aneroid gauge should be viewed straight on.

Discussion

A tight sleeve may act as a tourniquet on the arm or make it impossible to apply the cuff properly, which could contribute to an inaccurate blood pressure measurement.

Improper placement of the cuff can result in inaccurate blood pressure readings as a result of inadequate compression of the brachial artery or rubbing of the cuff against the stethoscope, producing noises that make it difficult to obtain a reading.

If the cuff is not applied properly, it may bulge or slip, and the pressure reading will be inaccurate.

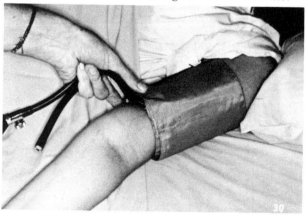

Correct viewing prevents inaccurate readings.

Key Steps

Discussion

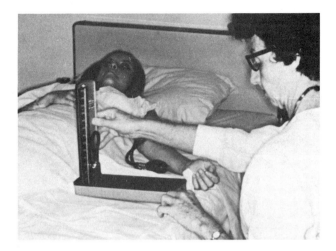

Place the earpieces of the stethoscope in a forward position in your ear canals.

With two fingers, palpate the brachial pulse at the antecubital space.

This position follows the normal anatomical position of the canals.

The brachial artery lies close to the surface at the bend of the elbow on the inner aspect of the arm and can be palpated on most people allowing optimal placement of the stethoscope to hear blood pressure sounds.

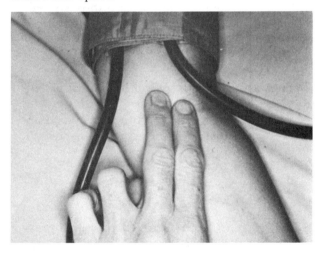

Gently, but snugly, place the diaphragm or bell of the stethoscope over the brachial pulse.

To hear all blood pressure sounds and hence achieve an accurate reading, there should be no gaps between the bell or diaphragm and the skin and yet no hard pressure against the arm to shut off the artery.

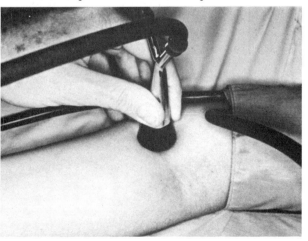

Key Steps

Discussion

Check to be sure the diaphragm or bell is not touching the cuff and that the tubing of the stethoscope is not touching or rubbing on anything.

The rubbing of any portion of the stethoscope on clothing or other objects will produce extraneous noises, interfering with an accurate reading.

Hold the stethoscope in place over the brachial artery with one hand, and with the other hand pick up the pressure bulb with a thumb and forefinger on the control valve.

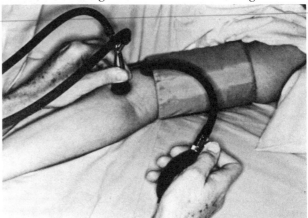

Close the control valve and pump air into the cuff until no sounds are heard through the stethoscope. Go 30 mm of mercury above that point.

When the cuff is inflated to the point where the cuff pressure exceeds the pressure of the blood in the artery, no sounds will be heard through the stethoscope because the artery is occluded.

Carefully open the control valve and slowly and evenly begin deflation of the cuff.

As you continue to steadily and evenly deflate the cuff, observe the gauge closely and note the following:

Blood pressure sounds are called the sounds of Korotkoff. The first sound heard through the stethoscope occurs when the pressure of the blood in the artery is equal to the pressure in the cuff.

- The point at which the first clear regular beat, the systolic blood pressure, is heard
- The point at which blood pressure sounds change in loudness and quality (first diastolic sound)
- The point at which the last regular beat, the second diastolic sound, is heard.

No further sounds are heard when the cuff pressure is less than the arterial pressure.

After the last regular beat, the second diastolic sound, is heard, open the valve screw wide, and completely and rapidly deflate the cuff so that the gauge reads zero.

If an immediate, successive measurement is necessary, wait at least 15 seconds.

This time lapse ensures that there is no compensation of the artery, which would interfere with an accurate reading of a subsequent blood pressure.

Immediately record the systolic and diastolic readings on a piece of paper.

Remove the cuff, and readjust the person's sleeve.

Cleanse the earpieces of the stethoscope with an alcohol sponge.

Prevents the spread of microorganisms from person to person.

Chart the blood pressure measurement, date and time obtained, and related observations.

Assessment of Peripheral Pulses

Objectives

The student will be able to do the following:

1 Discuss purposes for assessing peripheral pulses.

2 Locate four peripheral pulses in the lower extremities.

Introduction

Peripheral pulses in the extremities may be assessed to determine blood flow through the underlying artery or the condition of the artery. For instance, following cast application to the arm, the nurse might check the quality of the radial pulse to determine that the cast is not so tight as to occlude circulation. Persons with arterial insufficiency in the lower extremities need assessment of peripheral pulses of the legs. There are four common sites for determination of peripheral pulses in the lower extremities: the dorsalis pedis, posterior tibial, popliteal, and femoral arteries.

Procedure for Assessing Peripheral Pulses

Key Steps

Wash your hands.

Explain procedure and position person comfortably in supine position.

Assess pulses, starting at most distal artery and working toward heart. Compare pulses bilaterally as you move toward heart.

- Dorsalis pedis artery
  Palpate the middle of the dorsum of the foot between the first and second metatarsal bones. If unable to locate, palpate the entire dorsum of the foot. The position of the dorsalis pedis artery is quite variable. Palpating the entire dorsal surface ensures an accurate determination of the artery's patency.

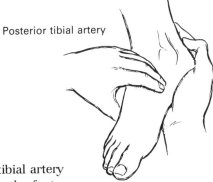

Posterior tibial artery

- Posterior tibial artery
  Dorsiflex the foot.
  Cup your fingers over the medial malleolus of the tibia so that the fingers slide off into the groove below this landmark. Use firm pressure.

Discussion

Prevents cross contamination.

Adequate pulse at distal sites usually indicates adequate blood flow to extremity. Establishes basis for comparison for alterations in pulse.

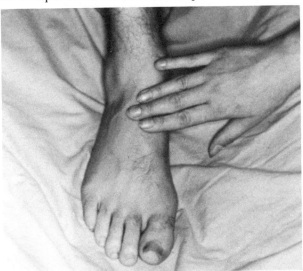

Dorsalis pedis artery

Facilitates feeling pulsations.
The posterior tibial artery passes behind and beneath the medial malleolus.

Key Steps

Discussion

- Popliteal artery
  Have the person lie in the prone position and cross the foot of the extremity being examined over the back of the other limb.

  Relaxes tissue in the popliteal space.

  Place fingers of one hand over popliteal fossa and press firmly.

  Popliteal artery is located deep in fatty tissue in the popliteal fossa. Deep pressure is required to feel the artery.

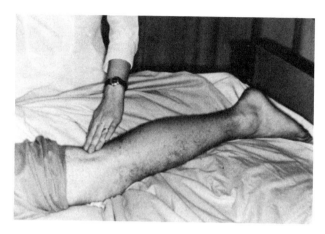

OR

Have the person sit down or lie in recumbent position.

Place your thumbs below the person's kneecap and the fingertips of your hands in the popliteal fossa (the indentation in the back of the knee). Feel for pulsations.

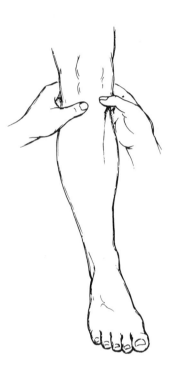

- Femoral artery
  Place fingers in the groin area below the inguinal ligament.

  The common iliac artery, which leads from the abdominal aorta, divides into the internal and external iliacs. The external iliac artery becomes the femoral artery as it passes beneath the inguinal ligament.

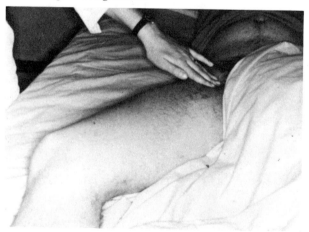

For each pulse obtained chart the quality and related observations such as skin temperature.

Promoting Venous Return with Elastic Stockings and Bandages

Objectives

The student will be able to do the following:

1 State the purposes of elastic stockings and bandages.

2 Apply elastic bandages and stockings correctly.

3 Recognize signs of impeded circulation from incorrect application.

Introduction

Elastic stockings are used to increase venous return by applying pressure to superficial veins and channeling the blood to the deep veins. This action prevents venous pooling and stasis, which are the major contributing factors in thromboembolitic disease. Elastic stockings also provide support for weak-walled blood vessels such as varicose veins. Finally, they prevent or reduce edema in the lower extremities. Elastic bandages are used for the same purposes and also can be applied to secure dressings and splints or to immobilize, support, and protect injured limbs and joints. If improperly applied, however, elastic stockings and bandages can impede circulation. The correct procedure must be followed carefully to prevent this from happening.

Elastic stockings and bandages should never be applied while the legs are in a dependent (below heart level) position. The extremities should be elevated or positioned at heart level (have the person lie supine) before application.

Procedure for Applying Elastic Stockings

Key Steps

Discussion

Check physician's order. One of three types may be ordered: full length, thigh length, below the knee.

Carefully measure the person for appropriate size and length. Measure both extremities.

Assures proper fitting so that appropriate amount of graduated pressure will be received.

Thigh length:

• Waist

• Length from waist to end of foot (posterior aspect of calcaneous)

• Diameter of thighs

• Diameter of calves

Full length:

• Length from groin to posterior calcaneous

• Diameter of thighs

• Diameter of calves

Below the knee:

• Length from posterior aspect of knee joint to posterior calcaneous

• Diameter of calves

Key Steps

Depending on manufacturer's instructions for measurement, the diameter of ankles may also be required. A special measuring tape for the extremity can be obtained, but this exacting measurement is rarely done by nurses.

To apply below-the-knee stockings, turn the upper half of the stocking over its lower half, and pull over the person's foot. Position the stocking over the foot and heel making sure the person's heel is centered in the heel pocket.

Pull stocking up to fit around calf. Smooth out excess material.

Discussion

Provides even compression and support.

Provides maximum comfort and prevents restriction of circulation that can occur with wrinkles and overlapping of elastic.

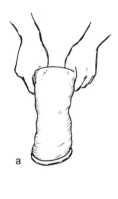
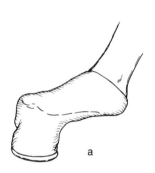
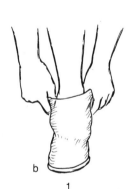
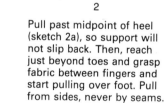
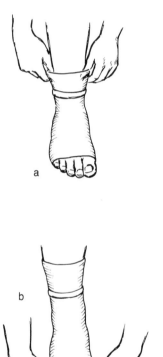
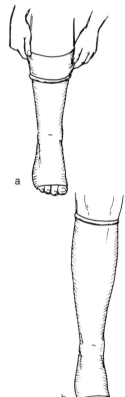

1

Sit with feet in easy reach. Support must be "inside out," with its foot inverted back to heel. Seam faces down (sketch 1a). Grasp each side firmly and pull onto foot (sketch 1b).

2

Pull past midpoint of heel (sketch 2a), so support will not slip back. Then, reach just beyond toes and grasp fabric between fingers and start pulling over foot. Pull from sides, never by seams.

3

Pull all the way up past ankle (sketch 3a). Seat heel in place. Pull foot portion of support out toward tips of toes (sketch 3b) to set fabric evenly on foot. Allow to settle back normally.

4

Using short (2 inches at a time), snappy pulls (sketch 4a), pull support up to point it was measured to end (sketch 4b). Smooth evenly down leg. Never allow top to roll or turn down.

Remove stockings at least 15 minutes every 8 hours to inspect condition of skin and check pulses. Observe warmth of skin and capillary refill.

Chart findings as appropriate.

Assures early detection of restricted circulation.

Procedure for Applying Elastic Bandages

Key Steps

Wash hands.

Gather the following equipment:
- Elastic bandages
- Clips or tape

Always apply elastic bandages from the distal to the proximal part of the body.

Apply evenly and smoothly, overlaping one third of the underlying bandaging. Spirals should be made diagonally on the leg rather than straight across.

Leave the distal portion of the limb exposed.

To apply elastic bandages below the knee, begin by using a figure eight wrap around the heel.

From heel, apply up the leg using a spiral or figure eight wrap depending upon the activity level of the person and the purpose for needing the wrap. The spiral wrap is most effective for use on persons with restricted activity or an immobilized limb or to secure a dressing.

The figure eight wrap is recommended for use with persons who are ambulatory or restless.

Secure ends of bandages with clips and tape, or just tape.

Discussion

Promotes venous return to the heart.

Prevents a "tourniquet effect" and uneven pressure on body surfaces, which can interfere with circulation and therefore with cell nourishment in the area.

Provides area for observing circulation. Promotes early detection of any restriction in circulation.

Secures bandage. Allows the bandage to bend when person is walking.

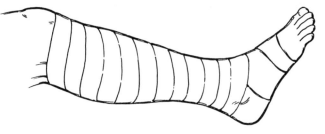

Spiral wrapping is easily displaced and wrinkled and thus less effective in providing even compression and support.

Figure eight wrapping is stronger and more reliable and thus provides even compression and support.

Prevents wraps from becoming easily displaced and thus interrupting even compression and support.

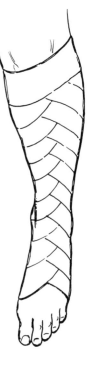

Key Steps	*Discussion*
Avoid using metal clips over bony prominences.	Prevents skin breakdown, which can occur with pressure and friction caused by clips.
Frequently check the circulation of the exposed distal portion of the limb (toes, fingers) while wrapping and afterwards. Signs and symptoms of restricted circulation are: blanching, cyanosis, tingling sensation, swelling, and coolness to touch. Immediate signs or symptoms of restricted circulation may indicate the wrap has been applied too tightly.	Assures early detection of restricted circulation.
Remove wrap for 15 minutes every 8 hours, and observe condition of skin.	Assures early detection of skin breakdown.
Check wrap frequently for wrinkles or displacement, and rewrap as necessary.	Maintains even compression and support.
Chart findings as appropriate.	

References

1. Sims-Williams A: Temperature taking with glass thermometer: A review. J Adv Nurs. 1:481–493, November 1976

2. Nichols GA, Kucha DH: Taking adult temperatures. Am J Nurs 72:1091–1093, June 1972

3. Nichols GA, Rufkin MM, Glor BA: Oral, axillary, and rectal temperature determinations and relationships. Nurs Res 15:307–310, Fall 1966

4. Geddes LA, Whistler SJ: The error in blood pressure measurement with the incorrect size of cuff. Am Heart J 96:4–8, July 1978

Respiration

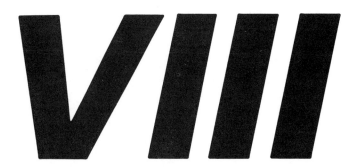

Environmental factors, disease processes, surgery, and immobility are examples of stressors that can affect the adaptive abilities of a person's respiratory system. In this section students will learn several interventions to assist the person to cope with altered respiratory function.

Nurses use physical assessment skills to evaluate the effectiveness of their interventions. When performing a respiratory assessment, auscultation of both the anterior and posterior thorax is done to determine normal or abnormal breath sounds. It is necessary to be able to identify the lobes of the lungs when auscultating (Fig. VIII-1).

Locating the Lobes of the Lungs

Using the location of bony structures in the thorax will assist in identifying the location of the lungs. In Figure VIII-2A, note that the apex of each lung extends ¾ inch to 1½ inches above the inner third of the clavicle. The sixth and seventh ribs are located at the lower border of the lungs in the anterior view.

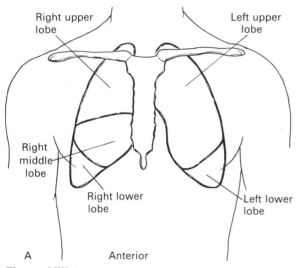
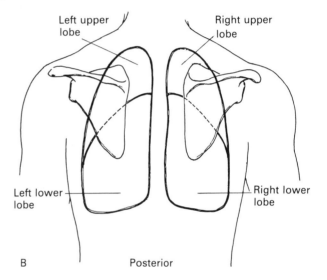

Figure VIII-1
Lobes of the lungs

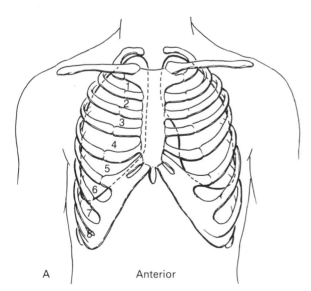
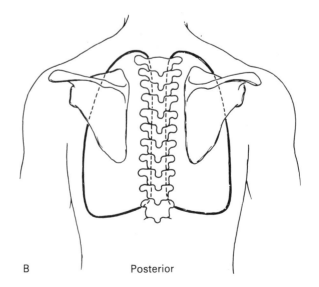

Figure VIII-2
Location of the lungs

143

In Figure VIII-2B, note that the lung apices extend above the scapulae in the posterior view. The seventh and eighth thoracic vertabrae are located at the lower border of the lungs.

Lung Auscultation

Before performing lung auscultation with clients, students should identify how normal breathing sounds through the stethoscope. There are three types of normal breath sounds: vesicular, bronchovesicular, and bronchial (Fig. VIII-3).

- Vesicular sounds are soft and swishing; the expiratory phase is nearly inaudible. They are heard over most of the adult chest. They originate from the alveoli.

- Bronchial (tracheal) sounds are loud, high pitched, and hollow. The expiratory phase is louder and longer than the inspiratory phase. Bronchial sounds originate in the trachea and are normally heard over the neck.

- Bronchovesicular sounds are somewhat louder than vesicular sounds; inspiration and expiration are equal in length and intensity. In the infant they are heard over most of the chest, but in the adult only over the second or third right intercostal space.

To perform auscultation of the lungs, assist the client to a sitting position, and ask him to breathe through his mouth slightly more deeply than normal. Place the diaphragm of the stethoscope firmly against the chest wall, beginning at the apex of the lungs and proceeding down alternating sides of the thorax, as indicated in Figure VIII-4. Listen to one full breath each time the stethoscope is placed, and compare one side of the thorax to the other.

Note areas of diminished intensity, recognizing that sounds normally diminish in intensity somewhat toward the lung bases. Also note any abnormal breath sounds. In the normal adult, only vesicular breath sounds are heard, with the exception of the right second and

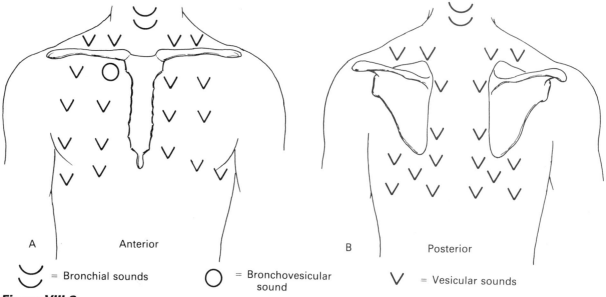

A   Anterior   B   Posterior

⌣ = Bronchial sounds   ○ = Bronchovesicular sound   V = Vesicular sounds

Figure VIII-3
Breath sounds

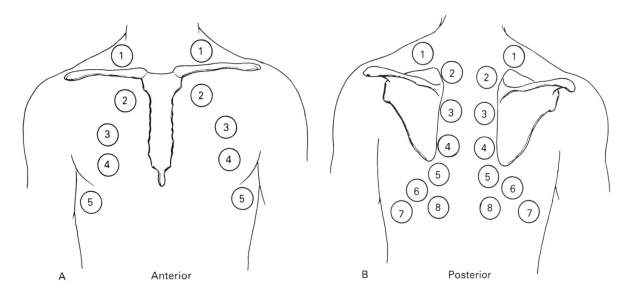

A   Anterior   B   Posterior

Figure VIII-4
Lung auscultation

third intercostal spaces where a bronchovesicular sound may be heard. Abnormally placed bronchial or bronchovesicular breath sounds indicate respiratory problems. Rales (cracking, bubbling sounds) or rhonchi (wheezing or snoring sounds) are also abnormal. See the accompanying text for a discussion of the significance of these sounds.

Coughing and Deep Breathing

Objectives

The student will be able to do the following:

1 Assist a person to perform coughing and deep breathing exercises.

2 Evaluate the effectiveness of coughing and deep breathing.

Introduction

Any person with increased respiratory secretions or decreased alveolar ventilation may benefit from coughing and deep breathing exercises. These exercises are often used for postoperative or immobilized patients. They are also used in conjunction with many of the respiratory therapy procedures described in this manual. For this reason the nurse should know how to assist the person to perform these exercises.

Deep breathing delivers increased oxygen to the alveoli. It also helps ventilate alveoli and promotes production of surfactant, which reduces the tendency of alveoli to collapse. Thus, deep breathing can prevent atelectasis. Coughing forces mucus from smaller air passages into large airways where it can be expectorated.

The person will cough and deep breathe more effectively in a sitting position. If he has an abdominal or thoracic incision it may be quite painful for him to cough and deep breathe. The nurse can help by holding a pillow, bath blanket, or hands against the incision while he coughs to stabilize it and minimize pain. This is called *splinting the incision.*

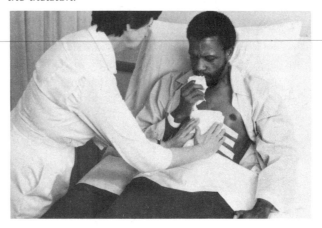

Procedure for Coughing and Deep Breathing

Key Steps

Assist the person to a sitting position. Place a pillow behind the person's head (not shoulders).

Auscultate the chest for the presence of secretions in the lungs. This will provide baseline data for comparing the effectiveness of the coughing and deep breathing exercises.

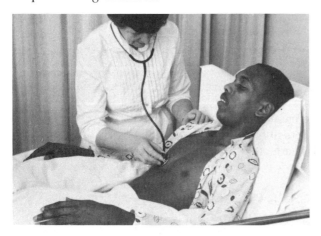

Instruct person to deep breathe as follows:

- Place your hands directly below the person's sternum in the "V" of the ribs so as to assist him to use the correct muscles when deep breathing.
- Encourage the person to push out your hands as he takes a slow, deep breath in through the nose.

Discussion

Ventilation is maximal in Fowler's position.

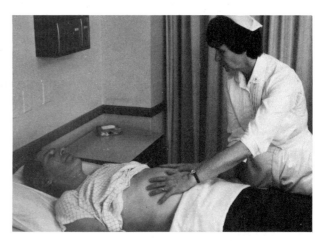

You should feel a gentle swelling of the abdomen under your hand, and the lower ribs should flare laterally.

Key Steps

- At the end of the inspiration ask the person to hold his breath for 3 seconds.
- Instruct person to exhale slowly and completely.

Splint incision with pillow or bath blanket if the person has an abdominal incision. This decreases incisional pain by providing support.

Instruct the person to take three deep abdominal breaths and end the last expiration with three short coughs.

Repeat the deep breathing and coughing cycle, depending on the person's tolerance.

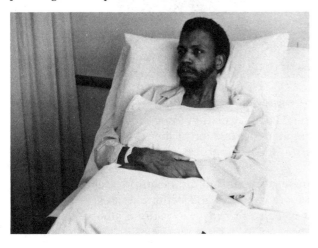

Auscultate the chest again, and note characteristics of the sputum.

Chart the frequency of procedure, description of coughing effect, whether sputum was raised, description of sputum characteristics, and auscultation findings before and after coughing.

Discussion

Sustains inflation of the alveoli.

Requires less effort than a single forced cough, and prevents airway collapse or spasm in persons with chronic obstructive lung disease.

Assists in achieving maximum effectiveness.

Checks for effectiveness of coughing up secretions.

Incentive Spirometer

Objectives

The student will be able to do the following:

1 Describe the purpose and indications for incentive spirometry.
2 Assist a person to perform incentive spirometry effectively.

Introduction

The incentive spirometer is a device that encourages deep breathing. There are many different models, but all work on the same principle. The person takes a deep breath through the mouthpiece of the spirometer. His effort is indicated in some way, for instance, by the number of balls he is able to raise in the spirometer or by the height of the ball in the cylinder (Fig. VIII-5). Because the person can see the effect of his deep breath, an "incentive" is provided that hopefully reinforces effective breathing.

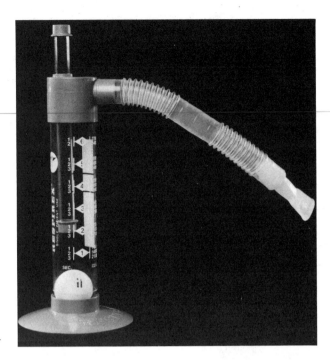

Figure VIII-5
Incentive spirometer

Spirometers are most frequently used for postoperative patients or persons on bed rest. Poor ventilation frequently occurs in these conditions. (See accompanying text for further discussion.) Deep breathing using the spirometer improves alveolar ventilation and prevents atelectasis.

Incentive spirometer teaching should begin preoperatively because the person is more receptive and better able to give a return demonstration. This will also provide a measure of the person's preoperative pulmonary ability, which can serve as his postoperative goal.

The procedure for using an incentive spirometer is usually initially taught by a respiratory therapist. A nurse must then assist the person to use it effectively.

Procedure for Using an Incentive Spirometer

Key Steps	*Discussion*
Assist person to Fowler's position.	Facilitates full lung expansion.
Instruct person to do the following	
• Exhale completely.	
• Place mouth around mouthpiece, and hold the spirometer level.	Ensures proper functioning of spirometer. If spirometer is tilted, the respiratory effort required to raise the ball is reduced.
• Take a slow, deep breath. This will raise the balls in the spirometer.	Expands the alveoli.
• Hold the deep breath for 3 seconds to maintain alveolar expansion for maximum alveolar ventilation.	
• Exhale slowly.	
• Repeat. Ideally, this should be done ten times each waking hour.	Maintains alveolar inflation.

Key Steps

Discussion

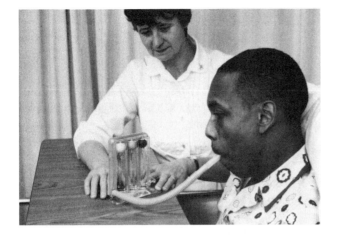

Check the setting on the dial of the spirometer. If the maneuver appears too easy, increase the dial setting. (Some models are equipped with a dial.)

Allow rest periods as necessary.

After each session, wash out the mouthpiece, and enclose the entire device in a clean plastic bag. (Manufacturer's instructions for some spirometer models may include washing the tubing.)

Incentive spirometry should be followed by coughing exercises to raise respiratory secretions, which can cause atelectasis or provide a medium for bacterial growth.

Chart the frequency of procedure and a description of deep breathing effort.

Increases required respiratory effort to strengthen respiratory musculature.

Prevents exhaustion and fatigue.

Removes microorganisms that may be a source of infection.

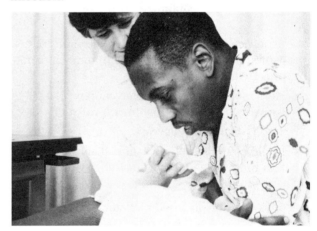

Tracheal Suctioning

Objectives

The student will be able to do the following:

1 Discuss purpose and indications for tracheal suctioning.

2 Perform tracheal suctioning using sterile technique.

Introduction

Some people with excessive respiratory secretions are unable to remove them by effective coughing, especially if they are very weak, have decreased level of consciousness with depressed cough reflex, or produce copious respiratory secretions (*e.g.,* in pneumonia). If the person is unable to cough and expectorate secretions effectively, mechanical suctioning of the tracheobronchial tree may be used. This procedure is unpleasant and is associated with several hazards including hypoxia, infection, and damage of tracheal mucosa. For this reason it is used only when absolutely necessary for prevention of airway obstruction and respiratory infection caused by retained secretions.

Tracheal suctioning may be considered a clean or a sterile procedure, depending on institutional policy. Sterile procedure is described here.

Tracheal suctioning is initiated with a physician's order, except in emergency situations.

How often should the nurse suction? Suctioning should be done only when needed, not on a "routine" basis. The following signs indicate that the person needs suctioning:

1 Moist, noisy, or gurgling breathing or moist coughing that does not clear secretions

2 Dyspnea or increased pulse and respiratory rate

3 Increased rales or rhonchi

4 Temperature elevation

Perform suctioning only when needed to decrease the incidence of the associated hazards.

Procedure for Tracheal Suctioning

Key Steps

Have the following equipment at the bedside at all times;

- Aspirator (suctioning machine). Pressure of the aspirator should not exceed 120 mm Hg to 150 mm Hg for an adult.
- Sterile whistle tip disposable catheter with Y-connector or thumbhole to control suctioning
- Sterile disposable gloves
- Bottle of sterile normal saline. (Label with date and time opened. Dispose after 24 hours).
- Sterile cups
- Stick-bag (for disposed catheters and gloves)

Wash your hands.

Explain the equipment and suctioning procedure. Assist the person to a semi-Fowler's position.

Auscultate the chest. Auscultation before and after suctioning provides a means for evaluating the effectiveness of the suctioning.

Discussion

Cleansing removes microorganisms that may be a source of infection.

Reduces anxiety and increases feeling of control. Semi-Fowler's position facilitates passage of the catheter.

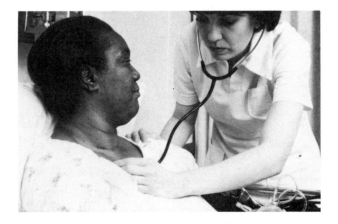

Key Steps	Discussion

Key Steps

Ventilate person with 100% O_2 if necessary.

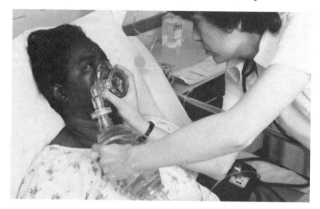

Pour sterile saline into sterile cup.

Select a #8 or #10 catheter. Open the package, leaving catheter inside package.

Open sterile glove and place on hand that will handle the catheter. Only one glove is needed.

Turn on aspirator, and pick up aspirator tubing with ungloved hand. Pick up sterile suction catheter with gloved hand. Attach catheter to aspirator tubing.

Using gloved hand, moisten catheter tip in cup of sterile saline.

Have person inhale. Introduce catheter through nose or mouth until cough is stimulated or resistance is met. (If going through nose, direct catheter straight back toward the ear.) Keep thumb *off* the thumbhole while inserting.

Discussion

Suctioning removes oxygen. persons with existing hypoxia, cardiac arrhymthmias, or compromised ventilation are very susceptible to the effects of suctioning-induced hypoxia.

Saline is used to lubricate catheter.

Allows access to the catheter when wearing sterile glove.

Only sterile gloved hand will handle sterile catheter. Ungloved hand handles unsterile equipment.

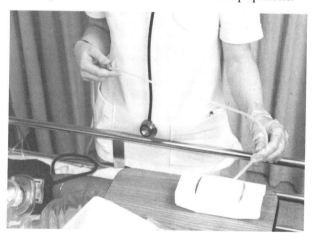

Lubricates catheter to reduce trauma to tracheal mucosa.

Avoiding suctioning during catheter insertion prevents trauma to tracheal mucosa.

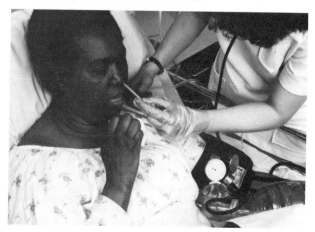

Key Steps

With gloved hand withdraw catheter while rotating it between fingers. Use thumb of ungloved hand over thumbhole to produce intermittent suction. (Thumbhole is now unsterile.) Suctioning should not exceed 10 seconds.

Discussion

This technique minimizes trauma to tracheal mucosa. Because suctioning removes oxygen, limiting time of suctioning minimizes hypoxia.

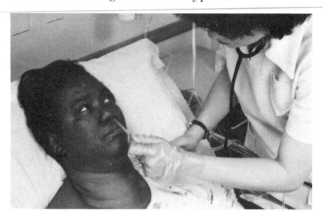

If the person vomits, suction immediately, continuing until the upper airway is clear.

Prevents aspiration of vomitus into the respiratory passages.

Aspirate saline from sterile cup through catheter.

Clears catheter of secretions.

Wait 2 minutes to 3 minutes before suctioning again.

Prevents hypoxia from continuous suctioning.

Repeat suctioning until secretions are cleared within person's tolerance.

Evaluates effectiveness of suctioning. You should hear fewer adventitious breath sounds and fewer areas of diminished breath sounds on auscultation.

Give emotional support throughout procedure.

Suctioning often causes severe apprehension.

Discard glove and catheter in stick bag. Discard cup holding normal saline.

Fresh catheter and saline should be used each time.

Give mouth care.

Reposition person comfortably.

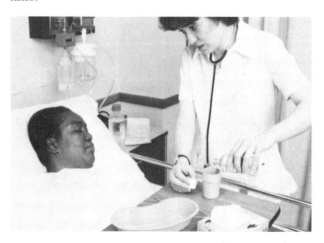

Wash hands.

Prevents potential spread of infection.

Chart the description of sputum, frequency of suctioning, description of auscultation findings before and after suctioning, and any abnormalities (e.g., bleeding or arrhythmias produced by suctioning).

Postural Drainage and Percussion

Objectives

The student will be able to do the following:

1 Identify purposes, indications, and contraindications for percussion and postural drainage therapy.

2 Perform percussion and postural drainage therapy using correct technique.

3 Evaluate the effectiveness of therapy.

Introduction

Postural drainage uses gravity to drain mucous secretions from small airways into larger ones where they may be removed by coughing. Postural drainage is used for persons with increased pulmonary secretions. If allowed to accumulate, these secretions could obstruct airways, causing hypoxia or infection. Common conditions where postural drainage is used include the following:

- Chronic obstructive pulmonary disease (COPD)
- Asthma
- Cystic fibrosis
- Pneumonia
- Postoperative states (usually only when there are unusually large amounts of secretions or ineffective cough)
- Comatose states

Postural drainage is contraindicated when cyanosis or dyspnea are increased by its use or when pulmonary embolus is suspected. It should also be avoided for persons with unstable vital signs or in untreated tuberculosis. Certain positions (*e.g.*, Trendelenburg) are contraindicated for persons with increased intracranial pressure.

Nurses can initiate postural drainage whenever they feel the person needs assistance raising secretion. Remember that any time you turn a patient, you are performing postural drainage!

Postural drainage therapy can be used alone, but it is often combined with percussion techniques. Percussion is rhythmic clapping over the chest wall with cupped hands. This technique loosens mucus in the lungs and is done over areas of pulmonary congestion.

Using the correct hand position is very important to prevent hurting the person. The fingers and thumb are held together and flexed to form a "cup" with the palm of the hand. See Figure VIII-6 for an illustration of the hand position for percussion. Avoid percussing over the breasts, spine, and kidneys.

Percussion is contraindicated over areas of carcinoma, in untreated tuberculosis, in pulmonary hemorrhage, and in pneumothorax. It should also be avoided if the person has a painful lung condition or a disease or recent surgery involving the chest wall.

Figure VIII-6
Correct positioning of hands for percussion

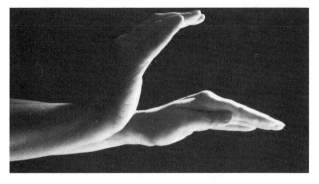
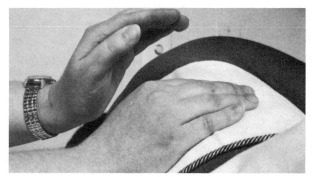

It is best to avoid percussion if the person has a recent history of seizures.

Percussion is usually begun only with a physician's order. Percussion and postural drainage techniques are often performed by physical therapists as well as nurses.

Percussion or postural drainage are usually performed three times daily. The best times are just before meals, when first arising, or at bedtime. Avoid doing either technique for 1 hour after meals because vomiting could result. If there is a physician's order for percussion, it should indicate how many times per day to perform therapy. The entire procedure takes 15 minutes to 30 minutes, depending on how many different positions the person uses. Treatments may be shortened and done more frequently if the person has difficulty tolerating them.

The positions to be used may be indicated by the physician. They may also be determined by the nurse based on the following:

1 Chest x-ray findings

2 Findings from chest auscultation

3 Prior knowledge of which positions produce the most sputum

4 Findings from palpation (Areas of congestion produce a "buzzing" feeling to the nurse's hands as the person forcefully exhales.)

The person may use one or more of the nine positions shown in Figure VIII-7. Percussion points are described in Table VIII-1.

These techniques may be performed at home or in the hospital. A family member may be taught to perform them at home. The person and his family need teaching about these procedures if he is to do them at home. Some suggestions for positioning at home include the following:

• Use wedge reading pillows or bolsters to lie across. They may be placed on top of a firm sofa pillow for additonal height.

• Use an ottoman with a soft pillow placed on top and lie across it.

• A child's bed or cot can be elevated at the foot on a box that is 16 inches high and filled to the top with newspapers. Push the head of the bed against the wall for safety.

Table VIII-1.   Percussion Points for Various Postural Drainage Positions

Percuss over the following areas (refer to positions shown in Fig. VIII-7):

Position 1: (a) Directly under the collar bones
(b) Above the shoulder blade; let your fingers curve over the top of the shoulder.

Positions 2 and 3: Directly over the shoulder blade

Position 4: Directly over the nipple or just above the breast (not over breast)

Position 5: Under the arm; let your fingers curve over the front of the chest.

Position 6: Over the midportion of the side of the chest

Position 7: From below the shoulder blade to the bottom of the ribs, not over the backbone

Position 8: From below the nipple line to the bottom of the ribs, not over the stomach

Position 9: Directly under the shoulder blade

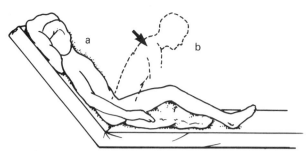

1 Upper lobe: (a) apical segment (anterior)
(b) apical segment (posterior)

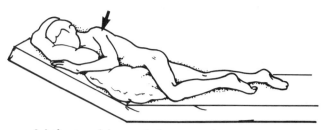

2 Left upper lobe: posterior segment

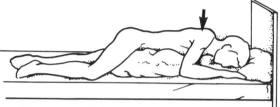

3 Right upper lobe: posterior segment

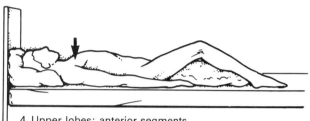

4 Upper lobes: anterior segments

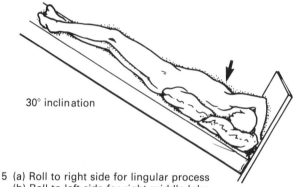

30° inclination

5 (a) Roll to right side for lingular process
(b) Roll to left side for right middle lobe

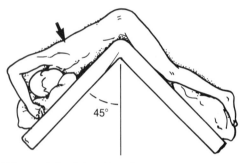

45°

6 Lower lobe: lateral basal segment
(a) Roll to left for right lower lobe
(b) Roll to right for left lower lobe

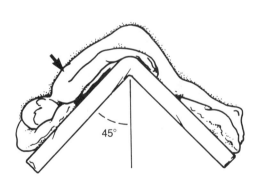

45°

7 Lower lobes: posterior basal segments

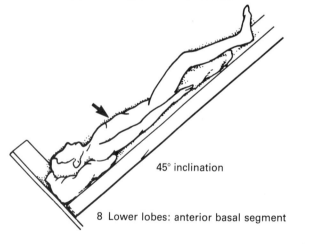

45° inclination

8 Lower lobes: anterior basal segment

9 Lower lobes: apical segments

Figure VIII-7
Postural drainage positions. (After
form from Division of Physical Therapy,
University of Michigan Medical Center,
Ann Arbor, MI)

Procedure for Postural Drainage and Percussion

Key Steps	*Discussion*

Gather the following equipment:

- Tissues
- Emesis basin
- Pillows
- Suction equipment (if person is unable to cough and clear his airway)

Orient the person to the procedure. — Elicits client cooperation and decreases anxiety.

Wash your hands.

If the person is receiving nebulized medications, these should be administered about 15 minutes prior to this procedure. — Promotes optimum loosening and expectoration of secretions.

Auscultate the anterior and posterior chest. This identifies areas of abnormalities (*i.e.*, rales, rhonchi, or diminished breath sounds) and provides objective baseline data.

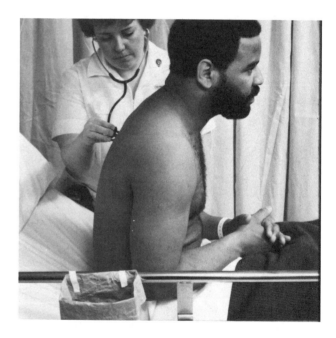

Instruct the person to use diaphragmatic breathing throughout the treatment. He should inhale deeply through the nose, *slowly* and quietly, letting the abdominal muscles rise. He should exhale through his mouth, a little harder and faster, contracting the abdominal muscles. Avoid "gasping." — Assists in obtaining full lung expansion for optimal alveolar ventilation.

Position the person in the desired postural drainage position. If necessary, use pillows to achieve proper positioning. — Promotes drainage from small pulmonary branches into larger pulmonary branches, using gravity assistance to drain secretions.

Percuss chest wall for 1 minute to 2 minutes using cupped hands and alternately clapping the chest with each hand. Areas for percussion are listed in Table VIII-1. Avoid percussing over the breasts, spine, and kidneys. — Transmits vibrations of air trapped in cupped hand through chest wall and into deeper lung tissue. Assists in loosening mucus, which tends to adhere to bronchi and bronchioles.

Key Steps

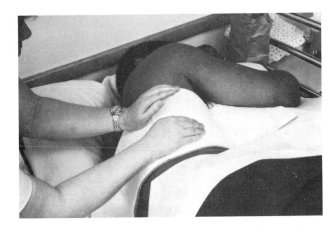

After percussing, encourage the person to cough (usually three times) so that loosened secretions can be expectorated and the passageways cleared. Have tissues and sputum receptacle readily available.

Wait several minutes, then repeat the percussion and cough cycle.

Change to a new position, or terminate the procedure when you note the following:

• Coughing produces no more sputum.

• Secretions can no longer be felt or heard.

• The person exhibits fatigue, dyspnea, cyanosis, nausea, or dizziness, or syncope occurs.

After therapy, auscultate the chest again.

Offer the person mouth care.

Chart percussion areas and postural drainage positions used, length of treatment, characteristics of secretions, findings of auscultation before and after therapy, and the person's tolerance to the procedure.

Discussion

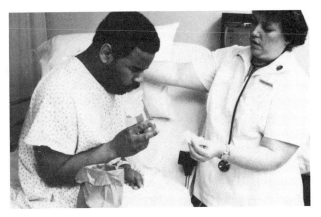

Provides rest period, which increases the person's ability to tolerate the procedure and yields enhanced effectiveness of secretion clearance.

Signals that indicate that areas of pulmonary congestion have been cleared or the person's ability to tolerate the procedure has been reached.

Identifies measurable changes following treatment.

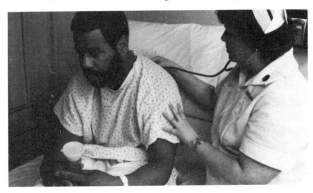

Provides hygiene and comfort.

Documents treatment. Provides accurate data base for comparison.

Other Considerations

Two additional procedures, nebulized mist therapy and ultrasonic therapy, are sometimes used for persons with increased respiratory secretions. Although they are usually performed by respiratory therapists, nurses should also be familiar with their effects.

Nebulized Mist Therapy

Nebulized mist therapy (NMT) is the passive inhalation of moisturized compressed room air. During an NMT, the person inhales and exhales independently, contrary to IPPB (intermittent positive pressure breathing) treatment, during which the person is forced by the delivery of gas under pressure to take a deep breath. If the person's room is not equipped with a wall outlet for compressed room air, a tank is used.

The normal saline nebulized mist is usually administered with an agent such as Bronkosol, which promotes enhanced alveolar ventilation by dilating the pulmonary airways. Mucolytics, which liquify thick secretions, or antibiotics may also be administered during NMT. To promote effective clearing of airways, it is essential that this therapy be followed by coughing and deep breathing.

Some conditions in which NMT may be ordered are: chronic obstructive pulmonary disease, pneumonia, asthma, atelectasis, and any condition in which ventilation is decreased or respiratory secretions are increased.

The most common hazard of NMT is an excessive elevation of pulse rate. It is for this reason that the pulse is monitored before, at regular intervals during, and after the treatment. NMT may need to be interrupted or terminated if the person's pulse rate increases beyond the limit specified in the institutional procedure manual. (The percentage of acceptable increase varies among institutions and is individualized according to the person's cardiovascular status.)

A physician's order is required for NMT. A usual order should contain the following:

1 Frequency (*i.e.*, q 4°)

2 Medication, if any desired (*e.g.*, Bronkosol)

3 Dose (*e.g.*, 0.3 ml)

4 Diluent (*e.g.*, 2.7 ml normal saline)

Respiratory therapists are usually responsible for administering the NMT, although in some settings, nurses perform this procedure. In any case, *both* the nurse and the respiratory therapist are responsible for charting (on a separate flow sheet or in the chart) the time the NMT was administered, the person's tolerance of and response to the treatment, and the characteristics and amount of secretions raised following the NMT.

Ultrasonic Therapy

Ultrasonic therapy is nebulized normal saline administered in a thick cloud of mist. This treatment is often ordered along with NMT. It is very effective in loosening thick secretions, making them easier to expectorate. For this reason, ultrasonic therapy is frequently used for sputum induction.

As with NMT, it is essential that ultrasonic treatments be followed by coughing and deep breathing.

Ultrasonic therapy administers a large volume of normal saline and can rapidly inundate the lungs with fluid. For this reason, therapy is contraindicated in pulmonary edema, congestive heart failure, and used with caution in persons predisposed to fluid overload.

Rest and Comfort

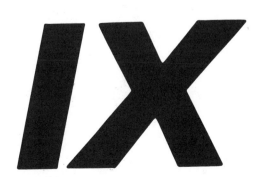

IX

In order to maintain a dynamic state of equilibrium and optimum health, each person needs to maintain a balance between rest and vigorous activity. Being able to relax fosters both rest and comfort. Rest and comfort in turn promote sleep, refreshing the person and renewing energy.

To determine the appropriate interventions, a thorough nursing assessment may be required to identify exactly what is contributing to discomfort or the inability to rest and sleep. A person-centered approach then suggests that the nurse will use a variety of strategies to facilitate rest and comfort. If, for example, a client is hungry, breathless, or feeling unsafe, these strategies will involve ensuring that those basic needs are met. A person-centered approach also suggests that the patient is assisted to use his strengths to attain personal control over his rest and comfort to the extent that he is physically and psychologically able.

Relaxation Techniques

Objectives

The student will be able to do the following:

1 Recognize appropriate situations for using simple relaxation techniques.

2 Use simple specific techniques to promote relaxation.

3 List common modifications, contraindications, and problems related to learning and using relaxation techniques.

Introduction

Relaxation involves soothing the mind and the body, specifically the muscles. Relaxation techniques are specific interventions or procedures intended to promote this relaxed state. The following are some purposes of relaxation techniques:

- To ease anxiety
- To diminish pain
- To increase comfort
- To ease contractions of skeletal muscle that may cause possibly painful stimuli
- To counter fatigue
- To alter vital signs
- To aid rest or sleep
- To improve response to other therapies

Relaxation techniques may be used for invasive procedures such as injections and aspirations, during pelvic examinations and dressing changes, and prior to diagnostic tests. From a holistic perspective, each person demonstrates an interaction between physical and psychological components. This interaction suggests more specifically a relationship between physical (muscle) tension and psychological (emotional) tension. The most nonspecific psychological or emotional tension is anxiety, as discussed in Chapter 15 of the accompanying text. Physiological tensions may include not only tensions of large skeletal muscle groups but also muscles under autonomic control. These smooth muscle responses include increased heart rate and blood pressure. The tensions of skeletal muscle are particularly amenable to control and relaxation by the person. Therefore, muscles are often the focus of relaxation procedures. It is thought that easing tension in one subsystem (physical) can ease tension in another subsystem (psychological) or *vice versa.* Thus, health professionals often advocate a combined approach to relaxation that includes both psychological and physical participation. In some specific relaxation techniques, certain forms of concentration or thought processes are also involved.

The particular relaxation techniques presented here are only examples of the many possible procedures that nurses can use. Once mastered through practice, these techniques are always at hand, ready for use in both acute-care and community settings. They may become one of your most commonly used nursing tools.

Procedure for Relaxation Techniques

Key Steps

Assess the person's need for use of relaxation techniques.

Determine the person's willingness and ability to participate.

Ask the person if he already uses specific technique(s) to relax.

If necessary, assist the person to begin technique as follows:

• Position person comfortably.

• Decrease environmental stimuli if possible.

Begin selected relaxation technique.

For moderate pain and fright:
Instruct client to do the following:

Discussion

Some considerations include the following:
• Are the person's muscles tense?
• Is he experiencing mild to moderate pain?
• Does he appear anxious?
• Is there restlessness or difficulty sleeping?

Any relaxation technique will be more successful if the person chooses to participate fully. Different relaxation techniques vary in the physical strength and abilities necessary for participation and also in the compatible personality characteristics and mental capacities.

Unless an emergency or severe pain prevents use, a previously learned technique may be preferable because it saves time or is personally satisfying. Builds on principle of conditioning a response.

Muscle tension is lessened in a position of alignment and support—slightly flexing joints lessens strain and pull.
Either a sitting or reclining position may be used.

Stimuli cause distraction and overload.

Key Steps   **Discussion**

- Breathe in deeply, and clench fists.

Purposely contracting muscles exaggerates existing muscle tension and enables person to perceive obvious contrast to relaxed state.

Active deep inspiration contrasts with passive, letting go of breath and enables long, relaxing expiration.

Deep breaths slow respiration and decrease anxiety.

- Breathe out, and go limp as a rag doll.

Expiration is compatible with relaxed muscles. Relaxing with expiration becomes a conditioned response.

- Start yawning.

A forced yawn leads to spontaneous yawning, which deepens and slows respirations.

For muscle tension in postoperative patients:
Instruct person to do the following:

- Drop bottom jaw slightly as though beginning a small yawn.
- Rest tongue quietly in bottom of mouth.
- Let lips go soft; breathe with slow rhythm: inhale, exhale, rest.

Muscles in this area may be tense as a result of intubation. Localized relaxation can promote generalized muscle relaxation. Requires minimal muscle effort and suitable for immobilized persons of diminished strength.

For anxiety and fright:
Instruct person to do the following

- Close eyes, and focus attention on breath.

Focusing on internal stimuli decreases perception of external stimuli that cause anxiety or fright.

- Breathe with slow deep rhythm.

Promotes muscle relaxation and decreases anxiety.

- Inhale saying "I am."
- Exhale saying "relaxed."

Talk is a form of conscious suggestion that client controls to manage anxiety.

Offer soft-spoken, positive encouragement.

Decreases concern over performance—trying too hard increases tensions.

Involve family member or significant others.

Use client's input to determine appropriate persons.

Instruct client to check for muscle tension periodically.

Slowing, flexing, extending, or rotating various joints gives biofeedback about how relaxed or tense associated muscle groups are.

Modifications

Relaxation techniques can be individualized according to varying needs, client preferences, severity of pain, prior abilities and relaxation experiences, and time and environment factors.

The specific relaxation techniques or interventions suggested may be used separately or in combination with other techniques, including meditation, autogenic training, progressive relaxation excercises, biofeedback, and mental imagery. Relaxation therapy is a more encompassing program that combines relaxation techniques with drugs, counseling, and physical exercise.

To help an infant or toddler to relax, hold the child in a comfortable, supportive position where the youngster may experience the nurse's rhythmic breathing and gentle comforting words. A rhythmic rocking motion may be helpful if not contraindicated. A slow, soothing, gentle rubbing motion or caress may be substituted if rocking is contraindicated.

Music may be a helpful aid to relaxation for those who enjoy it. Familiar and quiet music may be more relaxing than strange or robust music. Headsets not only keep music from distressing others but intensify auditory stimuli, which some persons may find helpful.

Daily practice for chronic pain results in conditioning.

The nurse should be alert to the possibility of undesirable side-effects, which may necessitate reassessment and altered interventions. For example, if relaxation techniques increase awareness of pain or body sensations, a mental distraction technique may be useful. Some body sensations such as tingling extremities are not unusual during relaxation. Assurance of their normalcy and possible repositioning may be useful. More serious possible problems include withdrawal, insomnia, and the feeling of suffocation.

Among the contraindications to using relaxation techniques are severe pain, the client's inability or unwillingness to participate, or specific physician orders against such.

Back Massage

Objectives

The student will be able to do the following:

1 Use touch to demonstrate caring.

2 Use massage techniques appropriate to person and purpose.

3 Record pertinent observations.

Introduction

Back massage may serve a variety of purposes:

- Promotes local circulation.

- Relieves muscle tension.

- Promotes relaxation.

- Enhances comfort through skin stimulation.

- Demonstrates caring.

- Provides for skin observation to assess general skin condition, edema, or pressure damage.

Several massage techniques may be used, depending on the desired effect of the massage. The following are examples:

- *Effleurage* is a stroking motion that may be deep or superficial. The hands move up the back with firm pressure on either side of the spine. Pressure on the spine causes discomfort, and the muscle mass to be massaged is adjacent and lateral to the spine. A lighter pressure is used across the shoulders and down the sides while the hands maintain skin contact. Long, slow, rhythmic strokes are soothing and may be used to promote relaxation. For example, this technique can be used during childbirth to produce muscle relaxation.

- *Pétrissage* is a kneading stroke. Grasp a large bunch of skin and muscle and move the hands up the sides of the spine and then across the whole back. Pétrissage feels stimulating and increases local circulation.

- *Tapotement* is a tapping motion that uses the ulnar side of the hand to percuss along the length of the back. Tapotement would not be appropriate for the very emaciated or debilitated person.

Several substances can be used to lubricate the hands, depending on skin condition, person's preference, and the purpose of the massage. Alcohol may be refreshing but dries skin and also may be harsh for elderly persons or the very young. Powder may be preferable to lotion in warm weather. Lotions and creams help retain skin moisture.

Procedure for Back Massage

Key Steps

Wash hands in warm water.

Bring a lubricant, powder, or alcohol to the bedside.

Place bed at comfortable height.

Move person on side or abdomen to edge of bed near you if not contraindicated.

Fold covers down below the buttocks, and drape the lower hip area.

Stand relaxed with good base of support.

Lubricate the hands.

Discussion

Hands should be warm before touching back.

Selection will depend on skin condition, person's preference, and purpose of massage.

Minimizes muscle strain and discomfort for the nurse.

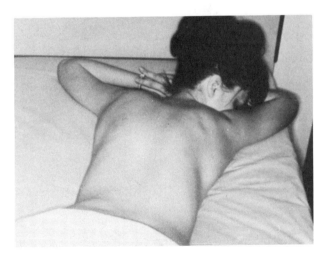

Discomfort may be communicated to person and may make nurse rush procedure.

Key Steps

Start with light stroking, keeping hands on back when changing strokes.

Use strokes suited to person and purpose.

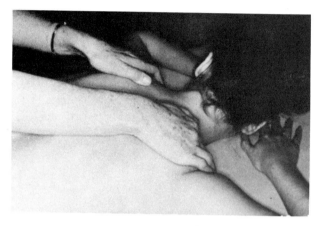

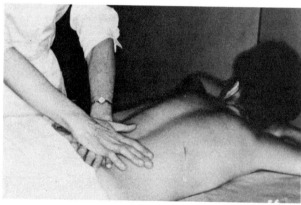

Encourage person to verbalize response.

Record responses and observations as appropriate.

Discussion

Helps to establish rapport and communicate caring. Short, quick strokes tend to be less comfortable than long, smooth strokes, which maintain skin contact.

Different strokes are intended for different purposes. Time will also be adjusted to suit purpose.

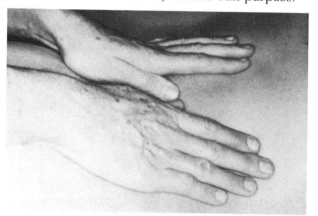

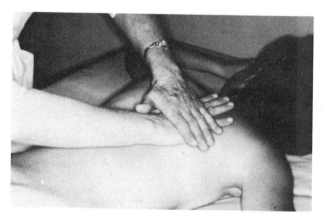

Was intended effect achieved? What modifications would increase person's satisfaction?

Medications

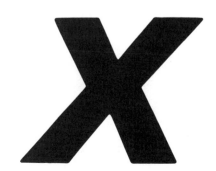

X

Medications may play an important part in the treatment of a person coping with illness or loss of functional ability. The nurse has many responsibilities related to anyone receiving drugs. These responsibilities include the following:

- Having an in-depth knowledge of the drugs that are being administered
- Obtaining drug histories
- Administering medications safely
- Observing and interpreting the person's response to medications
- Teaching persons about drug therapy

Within institutions, the drugs that are given are monitored carefully. Physicians prescribe some medications to be taken at specific times. Other drugs are available to be taken p.r.n. (as needed). Usually drugs that are taken at home are discontinued or collected unless specifically ordered by the attending physician. Rules vary with institutions regarding what medications may be kept at the bedside for personal use.

Drugs may be stored centrally for distribution or kept separately for individual persons. Regardless, the nurse is expected to follow a health-care agency's policy to avoid drug errors and drug abuse. Narcotics require especially careful monitoring to control drug abuse and to meet the requirements set by federal law.

To administer medications safely, the nurse requires knowledge of the approximate equivalents for weight and liquid measures and household measures (Tables X-1 through X-3) and other common abbreviations related to drug prescriptions (Table X-4). Additionally, the nurse observes the six "rights" of medication administration as follows:

- RIGHT PERSON
- RIGHT DRUG
- RIGHT DOSE
- RIGHT ROUTE
- RIGHT TIME
- RIGHT DOCUMENTATION

Table X-1. Approximate Equivalents for Liquid Measures

Metric (ml)		Approximate Apothecary Equivalents	Metric (ml)		Approximate Apothecary Equivalents
1000	ml	1 qt	3	ml	45 minims (m)
750	ml	1½ pts	2	ml	30 m
500	ml	1 pt (16 fl oz)	1	ml	15 m
250	ml	8 fl oz	0.75	ml	12 m
200	ml	7 fl oz	0.6	ml	10 m
100	ml	3½ fl oz	0.5	ml	8 m
50	ml	1¾ fl oz	0.3	ml	5 m
30	ml	1 fl oz (8 fl dr)	0.25	ml	4 m
15	ml	4 fl dr	0.2	ml	3 m
10	ml	2½ fl dr	0.1	ml	1½ m
8	ml	2 fl dr	0.06	ml	1 m
5	ml	1¼ fl dr	0.05	ml	¾ m
4	ml	1 fl dr (60 m)	0.03	ml	½ m

Common routes for administering drugs include the following:

- Oral
- Parenteral
    Subcutaneous
    Intramuscular
    Intravenous
- Topical
- Inhalation

Table X-2. Approximate Equivalents for Weight Measures

Metric	Approximate Apothecary Equivalents	Metric	Approximate Apothecary Equivalents
1 g	1000 mg	30 mg	½ gr
30 g	1 oz	25 mg	⅜ gr
15 g	4 dr	20 mg	⅓ gr
10 g	2½ dr	15 mg	¼ gr
7.5 g	2 dr	12 mg	⅕ gr
6 g	90 gr	10 mg	⅙ gr
5 g	75 gr	8 mg	⅛ gr
4 g	60 gr (1 dr)	6 mg	¹⁄₁₀ gr
3 g	45 gr	5 mg	¹⁄₁₂ gr
2 g	30 gr (½ dr)	4 mg	¹⁄₁₅ gr
1.5 g	22 gr	3 mg	¹⁄₂₀ gr
1 g	15 gr	2 mg	¹⁄₃₀ gr
1000 mg	15 gr	1.5 mg	¹⁄₄₀ gr
750 mg	12 gr	1.2 mg	¹⁄₅₀ gr
600 mg	10 gr	1 mg	¹⁄₆₀ gr
500 mg	7½ gr	800 mcg	¹⁄₈₀ gr
400 mg	6 gr	600 mcg	¹⁄₁₀₀ gr
300 mg	5 gr	500 mcg	¹⁄₁₂₀ gr
250 mg	4 gr	400 mcg	¹⁄₁₅₀ gr
200 mg	3 gr	300 mcg	¹⁄₂₀₀ gr
150 mg	2½ gr	250 mcg	¹⁄₂₅₀ gr
120 mg	2 gr	200 mcg	¹⁄₃₀₀ gr
100 mg	1½ gr	150 mcg	¹⁄₄₀₀ gr
75 mg	1¼ gr	120 mcg	¹⁄₅₀₀ gr
60 mg	1 gr	100 mcg	¹⁄₆₀₀ gr
50 mg	¾ gr	1,000,000 mcg	1 g
40 mg	⅔ gr		

Table X-3. Approximate Household Equivalents

1⅓ dr = teaspoonful	=	5 ml
2 dr = dessertspoonful	=	8 ml
4 dr = tablespoonful	=	15 ml
4 oz = teacupful	=	120 ml
8 oz = tumblerful	=	240 ml

Table X-4. Abbreviations Related to Drug Prescriptions

Latin	Abbreviation	English
Ad libitum	ad lib.	At pleasure (as desired)
Ante cibos	a.c.	Before meals
Auris dexter	A.D.	Right ear
Auris sinister	A.S.	Left ear
Auris uterque	A.U.	Both ears
Bis in diem	b.i.d.	Twice a day
Capsula	cap.	Capsule
Cum	c̄	With
	cc	Cubic centimeter
Diem	d.	Day
	d.c. or D.C.	Discontinue
	dr	Dram
Et	et	And
Elixir	Elix.	Elixir
Granum	gr	Grain
Gutta	Gtt	Drop
Gramma	g	Gram
Hora	h	Hour
Hora somni	H.S.	Hour of sleep
	IM	Intramuscular
	IV	Intravenous
	IVPB	Intravenous piggyback
	IPPB	Intermittent positive pressure breathing
Minimum	m	Minim (drop)
	mcg	Microgram
	mg, mgm	Milligram
	mEq	Milliequivalent
	ml	Milliliter
Nox. noctis	noc.	Night
Nihil per os	NPO	Nothing by mouth
	oz	Ounce
Oculus dexter	O.D.	Right eye
Oculus sinister	O.S.	Left eye
Oculo uterque	O.U.	Both eyes (in each eye)
Os	os or (o)	Mouth
Per os	PO or (o)	By mouth
Post cibum	p.c.	After meals
Pro re nata	p.r.n.	As needed
Post	p̄	After
	q.i.d.	Four times a day
	q.o.d.	Every other day
Quaque diem	q.d.	Every day
Quaque, quisque	q.	Each, every
Quaque hora	q.h. (q2h)	Every hour (every 2 hours)
Recipe	Rx	Take (thou); prescription
Semi, semis	s̄s̄.	A half
Sine	s̄.	Without
Si opus sit	s.o.s.	If needed
Statim	stat.	Immediately
	sub.q., s.c., or s.q.	Subcutaneous
	tbsp	Tablespoon
Tabella	tab.	Tablet
	tsp	Teaspoon
Ter in diem	t.i.d.	Three times a day
Tinctura	tr., tinct.	Tincture
	Tx.	Treatment
Unguentum	ung.	Ointment
	U	Units

Administration of Oral Medications

Objectives

The student will be able to do the following:

1 Pour stock medications correctly.

2 Administer medications safely, including stock medications and individually prepared doses.

3 Observe person's response to medications.

4 Document medication administration.

Procedure for Administering Oral Medications

Key Steps

Determine administration times for standing orders or p.r.n. oral medications. Organize work so that medications are given within 10% deviation of ordered time between doses.

Obtain the following information about the drug and person receiving it:

- Rationale for drug for this person
- Drug's usual average dose
- Expected action
- Untoward reactions or side-effects
- Appropriate route of administration

The following available information resources may be used for reference:

- Physician's Desk Reference
- Hospital Formulary
- Commercial drug references
- Local pharmacists
- Drug literature

If uncertain about a drug, dosage, or route, consult prescribing physician or nurse in charge.

Wash hands.

Prepare drugs safely. Follow agency policy for confirming drug order:

Unit dose system:
Validate that unit doses are correct as dispensed.

Stock medications:
Choose bottle of drug that matches medication card.

Discussion

Drugs given earlier or later than ordered time may be considered medication errors.

Confirms own knowledge of drug and person receiving it.
Ensures safe administration of drug.

Assures that medications are not contaminated and new organisms are not inadvertently introduced by way of drug administration routes.

Assures that correct medication and dosage are prepared.

Key Steps

Check container label three times as follows:

* When taking container from supply
* Before pouring
* When returning container to stock shelf

Discussion

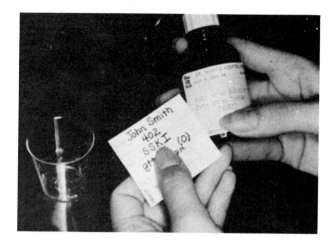

Pour medication directly into cup. Avoid touching medication with fingers.

Decreases possibility of contamination by microorganisms.

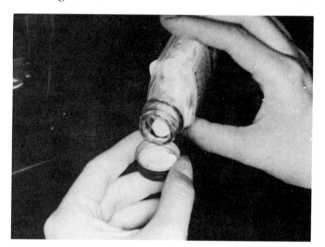

Transport medications safely:

* Keep drugs paired with correct medication cards. This assures that correct medication and dosage will be administered to appropriate person.
* Keep medications in sight.

Prevents loss or tampering by unauthorized persons.

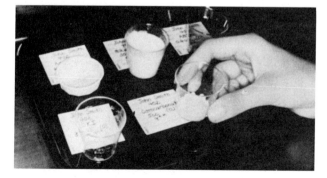

Key Steps

Discussion

To avoid administering the medication to the wrong person, identify the person as follows:

- Check arm bracelet and bed label.
- Ask for identification by person.

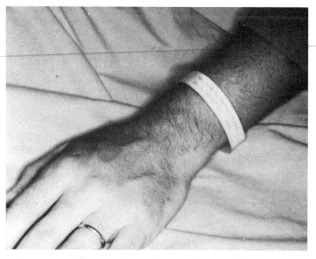

Administer medication as follows:

- Assist dependent person to sitting or lateral position.
- Provide water, and stay with person until drug is swallowed to confirm that medication has been taken.
- Juice may be offered with unpalatable medications if not contraindicated.

Assures safety and gravity assistance for swallowing.

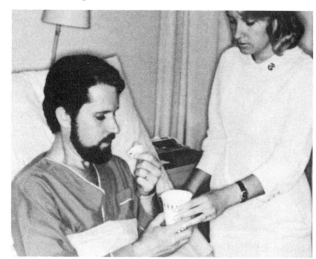

- Drugs that are irritating to mucous membranes may be diluted with fluid or given following meals.
- Certain drugs should not be given with milk, milk products, or meals (*e.g.*, tetracyclines).

Decreases irritation to mucous membranes and gastric lining.

Prevents interference of absorption of medication.

Chart according to agency policy. Full documentation includes date, time, drug, amount, route, and name of person administering drug.

Provides a legal record of drugs administered.

Modifications and Other Considerations

The administration of medications is often complicated by the number of persons the nurse must assist with medications. A system will be needed to organize the medication cards and to check cards for each person with the Kardex or medication book.

The importance of appropriate handwashing before the preparation and administration of drugs should not be underestimated.

Give only the medications that you have personally prepared unless a unit dose system is used. With unit dose, the medication comes already prepared in single-dose packets. The nurse dispenses these to appropriate persons. Nurses using unit dose need to be thoroughly familiar with generic names for trade-name drugs.

If the nurse must calculate dosage, the calculation is written and validated with another nurse if there is uncertainty.

Oral medications are withheld if person has npo orders (nihil per os or nothing by mouth). Oral drugs are also withheld if person is vomiting, unconscious, or unable to swallow. Usually the person who has a nasogastric tube for stomach or intestinal tract decompression will not receive oral medications. Drugs may also be withheld if the nurse's judgement indicates potential harm (*e.g.,* digitalis in a person with bradycardia). Check with the physician whenever you withhold a medication.

Hospitalized persons who have known allergies should have a caution sheet placed in a prominent place on their records. In the community, persons with allergies should be encouraged to wear special identification jewelry or to carry a warning card in their purse or billfold.

Various factors influence or modify a person's response to a drug therapy. Although most people respond similarly to a medication, many variables combine to affect individual responses, as in the following:

- The drugs the person is taking may offer a potential for additive, synergistic, or antagonistic effects.
- Certain drug side-effects may combine with the person's physiologic or pathophysiologic functions (*e.g.,* morphine sulfate in the person with altered respiratory function).
- Variations in age, sex, weight, and physical and emotional status influence drug effect.
- Persons develop tolerance to the effects of drugs over time.

Intramuscular and Subcutaneous Injections

Objectives

The student will be able to do the following:

1 Review sterile technique related to preparing and administering injections.
2 Select appropriate anatomical sites for subcutaneous and intramuscular injections.
3 Prepare medications accurately.
4 Inject medications safely.

Introduction

The nature of the prescribed drug or the person's condition may necessitate giving certain medications by injection.

With subcutaneous injections, only small quantities of medication can be administered (usually 1 ml or less). Absorption of medication is slow because the tissue is not very vascular. Therefore, subcutaneous injections are less than satisfactory for persons with inadequate peripheral circulation. Because there are pain nerve endings in subcutaneous tissue, pain is experienced on needle insertion and during injection of the drug.

Intramuscular injections are usually used for irritating substances in larger amounts but less than 5 ml. Absorption of a drug from muscle is more rapid because of the greater tissue vascularity. Muscle tissue contains nerve endings sensitive to pressure. Therefore, pain is experienced with needle insertion, and pressure is felt if the medication is injected too rapidly.

Anxiety or fear may be felt by the person anticipating injection. Gaining the person's understanding and confidence can decrease the anxiety and make a necessary procedure more comfortable.

Injections of any type break the skin barrier to infection. Using sterile technique decreases the possibility of introducing organisms into body tissue. Many agencies and persons at home use disposable equipment as one means of decreasing the infection risk.

To avoid the risks and discomfort of repeated injections, persons who require considerable medication that cannot be given orally may receive intravenous drug administration.

Procedure for Aspiring a Medication from a Vial

Key Steps

Discussion

Check label of vial with drug order. Compare dose with amount of drug per milliliter and calculated amount needed. Prevents error by ensuring preparation of correct drug and correct dosage.

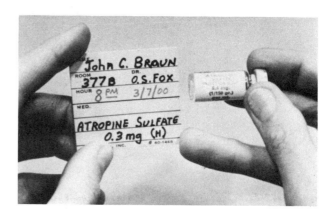

Select appropriate syringe and needle for intramuscular or subcutaneous injection. Must consider gauge and length of needle in relation to size of person receiving injection.

(See Subcutaneous Injections—Modifications, p 181, and Intramuscular Injections—Modifications, p 185.)

Ensures injection of medication into subcutaneous tissue or muscle mass.

Clean top of correct vial, using a disinfectant and friction rub on rubber diaphragm of vial. (Assists in decreasing microorganisms.)

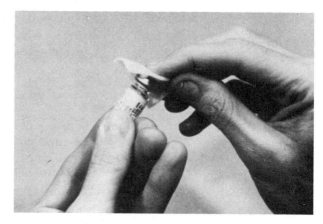

Remove needle cap, and aspirate amount of air equal to milliliters of drug to be withdrawn.

Most vials are vacuum packed so that drug withdrawn must be replaced with air to prevent plunger from being forced from syringe.

Key Steps

To decrease risk of contamination, insert needle with attached syringe into center of rubber diaphragm of vial, and inject air into vial.

Maintaining sterile technique, aspirate solution needed by pulling back on plunger of syringe, remove needle, and immediately replace needle cap.

Discussion

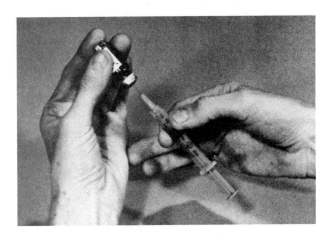

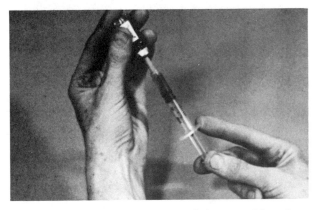

Recheck amount of solution withdrawn with calculated dose amount.

Prevents error by ensuring that correct drug and correct dosage have been prepared.

Modifications

Sometimes medications may be dispensed by way of glass ampules rather than vials. Remove the medication that has pooled in top of the ampule by holding it upright and tapping it with your finger. Cleanse the neck of the ampule with alcohol, and break off the top by quickly snapping the neck at the prescoring. Safeguard against injury to your hands by using a sterile pad or alcohol wipe when breaking the ampule.

Procedure for Subcutaneous Injection

Key Steps

Identify person.

Select a site, considering rotation if frequent injections are needed. Choose an area without large blood vessels and that is free of nerves. Rotation decreases tissue irritation and increases drug absorption.

Discussion

Prevents error by ensuring that the right person receives the injection.

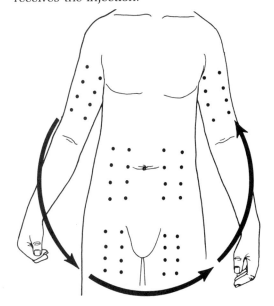

Key Steps	**Discussion**
Cleanse injection site, using friction and disinfectant.	The bacteria that normally reside on the skin are decreased to reduce infection.

Grasp and elevate subcutaneous tissue at injection site to prevent needle from entering the muscle.

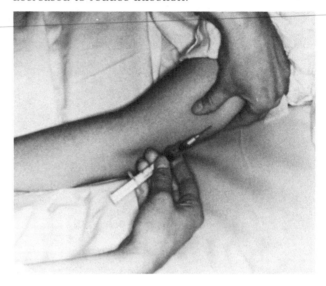

Insert needle at 30° to 90° angle.

Exact angle depends on amount and fullness of subcutaneous tissue.

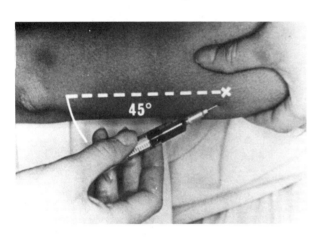

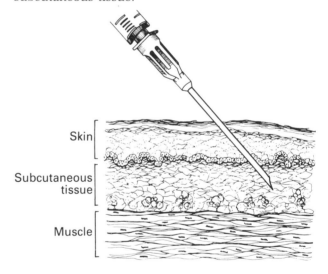

Aspirate plunger gently before injecting drug. If blood appears, gently pull the needle back and reinsert in a different direction. Check again for blood return.

Done to determine if needle is in blood vessel. Drug released into bloodstream might endanger the person as a result of immediate absorption.

Remove needle quickly, and rub area to decrease pain and aid absorption.

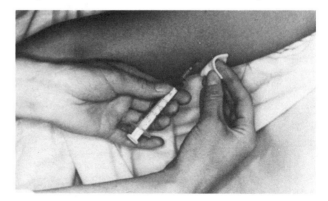

Key Steps	*Discussion*
Chart according to agency policy. Full documentation includes date, time, drug, amount, route, and name of person administering drug.	Provides a legal record of drug administered.

Subcutaneous Injection— Modifications

When the person is to give a self-injection, the site will be chosen for ease of self-administration.

Individual persons vary greatly as to the amount of subcutaneous tissue they have underlying the skin. The nurse needs to assess this individual difference before making a decision concerning the length of the needle and the angle of the injection; the following are suggestions:

1 For the average adult: 25-gauge, ⅝-inch needle at a 45° angle

2 For the very thin adult: 25-gauge, ⅝-inch needle at a 30° angle
There are also 26-gauge, ⅜-inch needles available that may be used for the severely dehydrated or emaciated person.

3 For the obese adult: 25-gauge, ⅝-inch needle at a 90° angle or a 1-inch needle at a 45° angle

Insulin syringes are often made with a permanently attached 27.5-gauge, ⅛-inch needle. Subcutaneous injections of insulin using these needles should be given at a 90° angle to assure administration into the subcutaneous tissue. Administering insulin to an obese person may require using a tuberculin syringe and a 25-gauge needle, choosing the needle length and angle most appropriate for the individual person. If using a differently calibrated syringe, remember to calculate insulin dosage accordingly.

Heparin, an anticoagulant, is usually administered in the abdomen at a 90° angle, 2 inches outside the umbilicus, using a ⅝-inch needle. Inject below the umbilicus where there is more fatty tissue. Areas above the umbilicus are used only if there are no other sites available. Avoid bruised and scarred areas. Heparin must be given as a deep subcutaneous injection to minimize local irritation, hematoma, and tissue sloughing. Heparin is injected using the "bunch" technique: grasp the tissue at the injection site, and create a "fat roll" about ½ inch in diameter. Do not aspirate or rub the site following the injection. This could cause a local irritation or hematoma. Gentle pressure may be applied at the injection site to prevent bleeding if necessary.

Procedure for Intramuscular Injection

Key Steps	*Discussion*
Identify person.	Prevents error by ensuring that the right person receives injection.
Select a site. The most common sites for intramuscular (IM) injection in adults are the following:	Always expose areas completely, and palpate each site.

Key Steps   **Discussion**

1 Deltoid

2 Dorsal gluteal

3 Ventral gluteal

4 Vastus lateralis

• Deltoid muscle

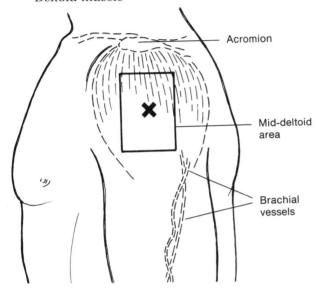

Offers ease of access regardless of person's position. Deltoid area available is limited when major bones, blood vessels, or nerves are avoided. Area cannot tolerate repeated injections or large amounts of medication. A line at the lower edge of the acromion process is the top of site. The two side boundaries are lines parallel to the arm, one third and two thirds of the way around the lateral aspect of the arm. The lower boundary is a line opposite the axilla.

• Dorsal gluteal muscle

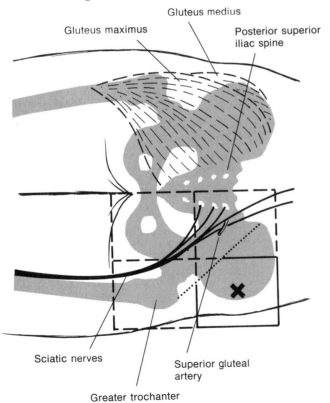

Hazards to avoid are the sciatic nerve and the superior gluteal artery.

Identify the greater trochanter of the femur and the posterior superior iliac spine. Draw an imaginary line between these two anatomical landmarks. Injection is given above and lateral to the diagonal line in the upper outer quadrant.

Key Steps	Discussion

Key Steps

- Ventral gluteal muscle

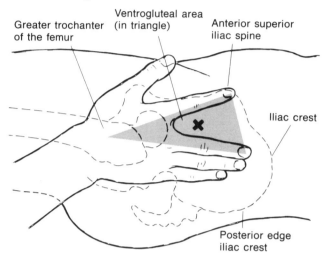

Greater trochanter of the femur — Ventrogluteal area (in triangle) — Anterior superior iliac spine — Iliac crest — Posterior edge iliac crest

- Vastus lateralis muscle

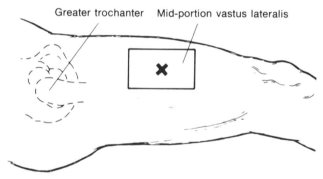

Greater trochanter — Mid-portion vastus lateralis

Position person comfortably. For example, to relax dorsal gluteal site, have the person turn toes in when lying prone. Injecting medication into a tight muscle can cause discomfort.

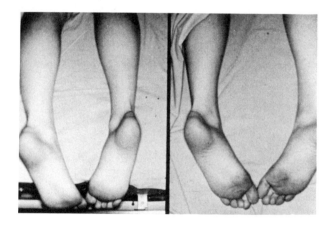

Cleanse injection site.

Discussion

When properly identified, site is free of major nerves. The index finger is placed on the anterior superior iliac spine. The palm of the hand is approximately over the greater trochanter of the femur. The fingers are spread apart, and the middle finger is placed ½ inch to 1 inch below the iliac crest, which the nurse palpates. The "V" formed by the index and the middle fingers outlines the site.

When properly identified, site is relatively free of major blood vessels and nerves. To identify the site, measure one hand's breadth above the knee and one hand's breadth below the greater trochanter. The side boundaries are the midanterior thigh and the midlateral thigh.

The bacteria that normally reside on the skin are decreased to reduce infection.

Key Steps

Discussion

Retract skin. Spread the skin taut with the thumb and forefinger of nondominant hand.

Taut skin provides a firm surface for easier needle insertion.

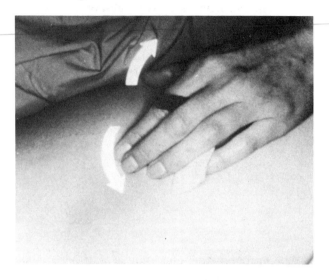

Draw an air bubble (0.3 ml) to cleanse needle and keep irritating solution from leaking back into subcutaneous tissue.

Insert needle, using a rapid darting motion with dominant hand.

The use of a sharp needle and rapid insertion will minimize pain.

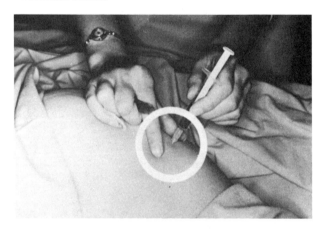

Aspirate plunger gently before injecting drug. If blood appears, gently pull the needle back, and reinsert in a different direction. Check again for blood return.

Done to determine if needle is in blood vessel. Drug released into bloodstream might endanger the person as a result of immediate absorption.

Inject drug slowly, remove needle quickly, and massage.

Decreases pain; massage of area facilitates absorption of drug.

Chart according to agency policy. Full documentation includes date, time, drug, amount, route, and name of person administering drug.

Intramuscular Injections— Modifications

A Z-track method of injection may be used if a drug is known to be particularly irritating to the subcutaneous tissue or if the drug will stain the skin (*e.g.,* iron preparations). After the solution has been drawn into the syringe, change needles. This will prevent tracking residual medication into subcutaneous tissue on insertion. Using your nondominant hand, retract tissue with the thumb and forefinger. Next, move your thumb forward and finger back, twisting the tissue. Inject the solution, but wait 10 seconds before releasing the tissue (Fig. X-1). It is important that the nurse select a needle long enough to pass through the adipose tissue into the muscle mass. The nurse decides on the basis of observation and palpation whether a short, medium, or long needle will be needed.

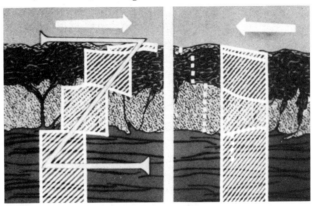

Figure X-1
Z track technique

To observe a site for the depth of adipose, gently lift a fold of skin and subcutaneous fat between your thumb and forefinger so that it is free of the underlying soft tissue and bony structure. The approximate depth of the subcutaneous tissue is one half the distance between the fingers. This technique is more difficult in the gluteal sites because subcutaneous tissue is closely adherent to underlying tissue. If an average person has ½ inch to ¾ inch of adipose over the site, add ½ inch so that the needle will reach well into the muscle tissue. If the deltoid muscle is used, a shorter needle is required than if the dorsal gluteal muscle is used, even in an obese person. If you are unsure of the length needed, having extra needles on the medication tray saves a trip back to the supply area.

Intravenous Therapy

Objectives

The student will be able to do the following:
1. Identify purposes of intravenous therapy.
2. Identify common sites for intravenous therapy.
3. Set up for an intravenous infusion.
4. Regulate intravenous flow rate accurately.
5. Change an intravenous container.
6. Identify complications of intravenous therapy.

Introduction

Intravenous therapy involves administration of medications or fluids into a vein using aseptic technique. The purposes of intravenous therapy are therefore as follows:

- To correct and maintain fluid and electrolyte balance
- To provide nutrition
- To administer medications

Medications may be given intravenously because of the following reasons:

- An immediate effect is desired.
- The drug is irritating to other tissue.
- It is important to maintain a constant blood level of a medication.

Common sites for intravenous infusion are the following:

- The forearm
- The upper arm
- Dorsal surface of the hand
- The antecubital space at the elbow

The forearm is a desirable site because it permits the person more freedom of movement and offers less risk of infiltration and other complications. Veins in the lower extremities are seldom used because of the danger of thrombophlebitis. The subclavian vein is a central vessel that is being used with increased frequency. The conditions for which the subclavian vein is chosen for intravenous therapy are the following:

- When providing parenteral nutrition is a main goal of intravenous therapy
- If monitoring of central venous pressure is desired
- If long-term therapy poses risks to smaller vessels

A subclavian placement requires a small incision near the clavicle. A tiny catheter called an intracath is then threaded into place. The risk of vessel damage is diminished at insertion but increased along the vessel, especially when intracaths are used in smaller vessels.

Nurses who care for persons receiving IV therapy will observe the following:

- The person
- Infusion site
- Tubing
- Flow rate
- Bottle or bag

Specific observations to be made are addressed in the procedure as appropriate. Also addressed are the observations related to preventing complications of IV therapy. Before beginning this section, students should review principles of surgical asepsis, because IV therapy is administered using sterile technique.

Physical care of the person with an IV requires special attention to such activities as changing positions and assisting in ambulation to prevent dislodging the needle or altering the intravenous flow.

Because providing emotional support is an important part of caring for the person's physical condition, all explanations are given with sensitivity to the person's unique needs and concerns.

Procedure for Setting Up for an Intravenous Infusion

Key Steps

Familiarize yourself with equipment.

- Needles

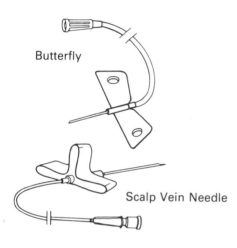

Discussion

Needle types, lengths, and gauges vary. Choice depends on characteristics of the person (*e.g.,* venous system condition and mobility) and the solution (*e.g.,* viscosity). The smaller the number, the larger the opening.

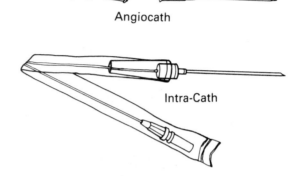

- Solution reservoirs

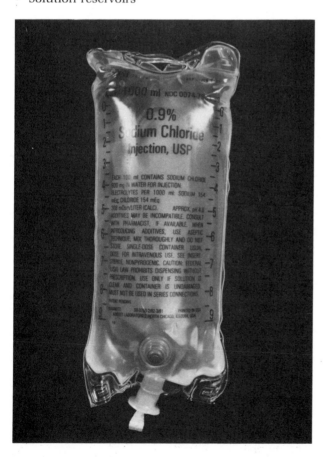

IV bottles and plastic IV bags come in various sizes and types. Note the following:

- Calibrations on solution container to indicate amount of solution used
- Where IV tubing inserts
- Where medications are added (medication portal)

Key Steps	Discussion

Key Steps

• Tubing

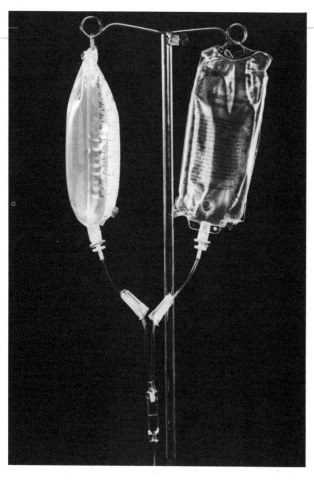

Prepare IV infusion set as follows:
• Check order carefully.

• Identify IV solution needed, and inspect bag for flaws, cloudiness, or foreign matter.

• Identify tubing needed.

• Insert tubing into IV container. Do not touch tip of tubing or bottle top or other surface.
• Expel all air (called purging or priming tubing).

Prepare person for infusion.

Position person for access to venipuncture site.

Discussion

Straight tubing allows only one container to be directly connected to person.

Y tubing allows two containers to be connected to person. When this tubing is used, one container is infusing, and the other is ready to be switched on when needed.

Tubing with extra length or a stopcock, which allows solution to run in three directions, may be needed in certain circumstances.

Note: drip chambers vary also. Regular type allows larger drops (e.g., 15/ml; mini-drip chamber creates smaller drops (e.g., 60/ml). Exact rate varies with manufacturer. Blood filter chambers prevent large blood particles from entering person.

Physician's written order must agree with IV card.

Read label carefully, checking that IV solution in container is *exactly* the same as ordered. If inspection of bag reveals flaws, cloudiness, or foreign matter, *do not use.*

Select the appropriate tubing based on anticipated need.

Maintain sterile technique.

Open clamp, and allow solution to run through tubing until all air is removed to avoid danger of air embolism. Squeeze and release drip chamber to fill it half way.

Explanation, emotional support, and comfort measures will vary, depending on individual needs of the person.

Procedure may be done by a physician or nurse, depending on institutional policy.

Procedure for Flow Rate Regulation

Key Steps	*Discussion*
Determine flow rate.	The flow rate often must be calculated from the physician's order. Usually the order indicates the amount of solution to be infused over a specific number of hours. The nurse calculates the rate in drops per minute (gtts/min). The following formula can be used to calculate this rate:

$$\frac{\text{Number of gtts/ml} \times \text{amount of solution}}{\text{Time in minutes}}$$

Example:

$$\frac{15 \text{ gtts/ml} \times 1000 \text{ ml}}{8 \text{ hrs} \times 60 \text{ min/hr}} = \frac{15{,}000 \text{ gtts}}{480 \text{ mins}} = 31\text{–}32 \text{ gtts/min}$$

Note, drops per ml vary according to type of tubing used.

An alternate method of calculating steps:

1 Divide total number of ml by the time in hours as follows:

$$\frac{\text{Amount of solution in ml}}{\text{Time in hours}} = \text{ml/hr}$$

This figure can be used when marking the bag (will be explained later in the program).

2 Divide the ml/hr by 60 minutes as follows:

$$\frac{\text{ml/hr}}{60 \text{ min/hr}} = \text{ml/min}$$

Multiply the ml/min by the number of gtts/ml delivered by the infusion set you are using as follows:

$$\text{ml/min} \times \text{gtts/ml} = \text{gtts/min}$$

This figure can be used when you are regulating the flow rate.

Keep-Open (K-O) Rate
When a patient has an IV for the primary purpose of keeping an open route for the administration of IV medications or blood, the physician will often order IV fluid to be administered at a "keep open" (K-O) rate. This means to regulate the IV just fast enough to keep it patent. Some hospitals have a standard K-O rate such as 50 ml/hr.

Time tape the container.

This manuever allows immediate determination of how much IV fluid has entered the person at a particular time. The tape should include the following:

- Time and date IV fluid began running
- Time IV solution should be finished

Key Steps

Discussion

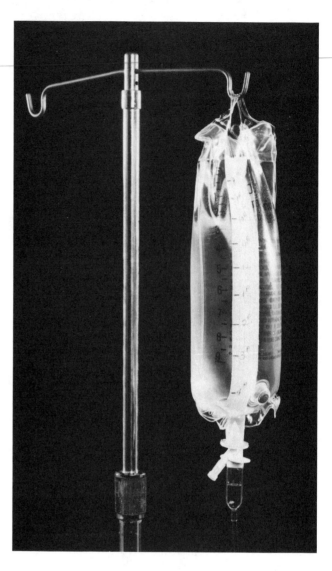

Monitor the flow rate.

Frequent adjustments may be necessary. To determine how quickly the solution is running, count the drops as they fall into the drip chamber for 15 seconds, and multiply by 4. Rate is dependent on fluid pressure in the delivery system and resistance in the person's vein. Fluid pressure is affected by the following:

- Height of fluid column
- Tube diameter
- Fluid viscosity

Vein resistance is affected by the following:

- Status of peripheral vascular system
- Vein diameter
- Needle position within vein

Key Steps	Discussion
	The many factors affecting flow rate make it necessary to monitor all persons at least every hour, and in some persons as frequently as every 15 minutes.

Procedure for Changing an IV Container

Key Steps

Discussion

Intravenous therapy usually involves the infusion of more than one container of solution. Containers should be changed before they become completely empty.

Avoids having drip chamber empty, which will prevent air from entering the tubing.

Prepare IV container.

Identify solution needed, inspect, and time-tape the container.

Take new IV container to person's bedside, and explain the procedure.

The need for explanations and support will vary. The person may be familiar with procedure at this time.

For bags do the following:
- Remove tear-off tab or cap from administration port of new IV bag, and hang new bag on IV pole.
- Remove old IV bag from IV pole, which is still connected to tubing.
- Remove piercing pin from old IV bag by allowing the old bag to bend, keeping drip chamber in upright position.
- Insert piercing pin into administration port of new bag that is hanging on pole.

Maintain sterile technique by not touching the administration port.

The old bag will bend easily now that it is nearly empty. This will prevent the remaining solution from pouring out. Maintaining drip chamber in upright position will prevent air from entering tubing.

Having the new bag hanging facilitates the maneuver of piercing through the administration port.

For bottles, do the following:
- Place new bottle upright on a flat surface, and remove cap or pull off tab. Clean top with an alcohol swab.
- Remove old bottle from IV pole. Remove piercing pin from old bottle. Quickly insert into new bottle, being careful not to squeeze drip chamber.
- Hang new bottle on IV pole.

Maintain sterile technique during procedure. Avoid squeezing to prevent emptying drip chamber, which would allow air to enter tubing.

Nurse may need to add solution to drip chamber.

Flow into drip chamber has been interrupted during container change, but infusion into person has continued, thus decreasing amount of solution into drip chamber.

Check flow rate.

Hanging a new IV container generally does not alter flow rate.

Key Steps	Discussion
Observe for complications at infusion site.	Possible complications include infiltration at needle site, inflammation, and thrombosis.
Chart amount and type of solution, route (IV), and time hung.	Provides legal record of solution administered.

Procedure for Ongoing Care in Intravenous Therapy

Key Steps	Discussion
Observe for complications, including the following:	
• Infiltration of needle	Site may be tender, firm, and puffy, indicating needle has slipped from vein and IV fluid is filling tissue around vein. If needle is in vein, lowering the container below vein level will cause blood to flow into needle.
• Inflammation	Redness, warmth, and pain at needle site and vein path may indicate phlebitis.
• Thrombosis	Infection, overuse of vessel, hypertonic solutions, and lack of blood flow along vein may contribute to clot formation. Also, if fluid flow stops, a clot will form.
• Air embolism	Air entering the vein can cause sudden dyspnea, cyanosis, collapse, and unconsciousness. A large amount could cause death. To prevent air embolism, do the following: • Make sure connections fit. • Use tubing without defect. • Check that tubing below drip chamber is completely filled with solution before infusion starts. This prevents infusion of air. • Change bottles before they are completely dry. Remember also, there must be solution above air in tubing to force air into vein; otherwise a clot will form.
• Circulatory overload	May occur even if IV is running at ordered rate. Elderly persons and children or those with renal and cardiac disease are particularly susceptible. Be alert for increased venous pressure, tachycardia, dyspnea, cyanosis, chest discomfort, and moist lung sounds.
• Infection	May occur from contaminated fluid or inadequate technique in setting up infusion or changing solution containers.
Assist person with activities of daily living as necessary	IVs placed in the arm may restrict mobility of extremity and impede ability to do ADL.

Key Steps	*Discussion*
Each time a new container is hung, chart amount and type of solution, route (IV), and time.	Provides a legal record of drugs administered; certain required documentation is basic, although institutional policies vary.

Other Considerations

Administering intravenous medications and use of infusion regulators are two other procedures that are related to intravenous therapy. Because the equipment and techniques vary greatly between institutions, only a general discussion is provided here.

Infusion Regulators

There are a variety of infusion regulators available to assist in the delivery of IVs. They are being used with increased frequency and in a variety of situations. Infusion regulators are generally used in the following situations:

- Infusions requiring very high or very low flow rates
- Infusions where extremely viscous solutions must be run
- Infusions of medications where extreme accuracy of amount and rate must be ensured

There are two basic types of infusion regulators:

- IV controllers—manage the force of gravity to obtain accurate and consistent flow rates.
- IV infusion pumps—create a positive pressure to obtain accurate and consistent flow rates.

The greatest advantage of an IV infusion regulator is its ability to deliver IV medications and solutions into the vascular system within a small percentage of the rate specified.

Infusion regulators are also advantageous because they are equipped with a sensitive alarm system. This alarm will activate and alert the nurse when certain problems occur, including the following:

- Empty IV bag or bottle
- Occluded or kinked IV tubing
- Positional IVs
- Deviations from the preselected drop rate
- Infiltrated IVs

The set-up, operation, features, and controls of IV infusion regulators vary among manufacturers.

Intravenous Medications

Medications are often administered by way of the intravenous route. They can be given in a variety of ways, including the following:

- IV push medications
- Additives to the primary IV
- Piggyback (IVPB) medications

The IV push method is used for drugs that are injected directly into the bloodstream. The person may or may not be receiving a concurrent IV infusion. Nursing responsibilities and special techniques for this type of administration vary among institutions.

A medication is administered as an additive to the primary IV when a continuous rate is desired. Medications are injected into the IV container through the additive port.

The piggyback method is used when medications are to be infused in a relatively short period of time at spaced intervals. IVPB administration causes an intermittent, rapid increase in the blood level of a medication. Antibiotics are a class of drugs that are commonly administered by this route. A patent IV infusion is necessary to allow for intermittent piggyback infusions. The piggyback medication is diluted in a burette, which is attached to an IV. The flow of solution from the primary IV infusion is temporarily stopped or slowed to a K-O rate while the piggyback medication is infusing (Fig. X-2).

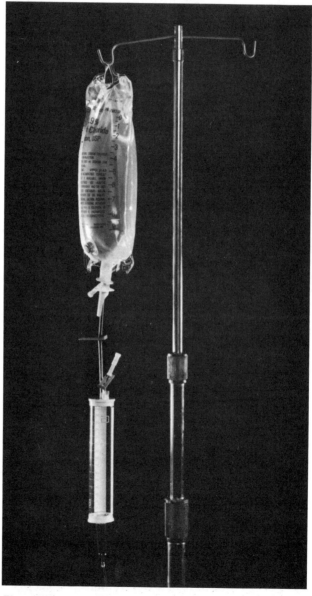

Figure X-2
"Piggyback" IV medication

General Summary

Scheduling Medications

Drugs requiring a constant blood level are usually scheduled evenly over a 24-hour period, for example, 6 am, 12 noon, 6 pm, 12 midnight instead of 8 am, 12 noon, 6 pm, 10 pm. These drugs include the following:

- Anticonvulsants
- Steroids
- Antibiotics
- Tranquilizers
- Blood pressure and heart drugs
- Antihistamines

Medication Dosages

Prescribed dosage of medications varies according to many circumstances and the individual characteristics of unique persons. These include: age, weight, sex, route of administration, the general condition of the person, and drug sensitivities or intolerances. Various formulae are sometimes used to determine reduction in adult doses appropriate for children of different ages or weights.

Other Routes of Administration

Medications may also be administered topically to the skin, as instillations into the ear or eye, or as rectal or vaginal suppositories. Topical medications are usually administered for their localized effect on the skin, although systemic action can occur. Use a clean glove, an applicator, or a tongue blade to apply the medication to avoid receiving the medication yourself. Be sure to follow any specific directions ordered by the physician, such as covering the medicated area with an occlusive dressing.

To administer eye drops, instruct the person to look upward and use your finger to gently pull down on the lower lid. Squeeze the prescribed number of drops into the lower lid, and ask the person to close the eye. Blot any solution that drains from the eye with a tissue. To administer ear drops, position the person lying on the unaffected side, or sitting with head tilted toward unaffected side. In adults, with your thumb and forefinger, pull gently upward and backward on the pinna. In children, pull downward and backward. Instill the prescribed number of drops, directing the medication toward the ear canal. Never use a container of eye or ear medications for more than one person.

Suppositories are lubricated with water-soluble jelly before administration. Lubricate only the tip of the suppository for easier handling. Introduce a rectal suppository with a gloved finger beyond the internal sphincter while the person is in a side-lying position. Vaginal suppositories are usually inserted in an applicator and placed high into the vagina while the woman is in a lithotomy position. Some persons may prefer to insert their own suppositories.

Index

Numerals followed by an *f* indicate a figure; *t* following a page number indicates tabular material.